Obstetrics and Gynecology: Maintenance of Knowledge

Editors

JANICE L. BACON
PAUL G. TOMICH

OBSTETRICS AND GYNECOLOGY CLINICS OF NORTH AMERICA

www.obgyn.theclinics.com

Consulting Editor
WILLIAM F. RAYBURN

June 2017 • Volume 44 • Number 2

ELSEVIER

1600 John F. Kennedy Boulevard • Suite 1800 • Philadelphia, Pennsylvania, 19103-2899

http://www.theclinics.com

OBSTETRICS AND GYNECOLOGY CLINICS OF NORTH AMERICA Volume 44, Number 2
June 2017 ISSN 0889-8545, ISBN-13: 978-0-323-53019-4

Editor: Kerry Holland
Developmental Editor: Kristen Helm

Obstetrics and Gynecology Clinics (ISSN 0889-8545) is published quarterly by Elsevier Inc., 360 Park Avenue South, New York, NY 10010-1710. Months of issue are March, June, September, and December. Periodicals postage paid at New York, NY, and additional mailing offices. Subscription price per year is $301.00 (US individuals), $627.00 (US institutions), $100.00 (US students), $377.00 (Canadian individuals), $792.00 (Canadian institutions), $225.00 (Canadian students), $459.00 (international individuals), $792.00 (international institutions), and $225.00 (international students). To receive student/resident rate, orders must be accompanied by name of affiliated institution, date of term, and the signature of program/residency coordinator on institution letterhead. Orders will be billed at individual rate until proof of status is received. Foreign air speed delivery is included in all *Clinics* subscription prices. All prices are subject to change without notice. POSTMASTER: Send address changes to *Obstetrics and Gynecology Clinics*, Elsevier Health Sciences Division, Subscription Customer Service, 3251 Riverport Lane, Maryland Heights, MO 63043. **Customer Service: Telephone: 1-800-654-2452 (U.S. and Canada); 314-447-8871 (outside U.S. and Canada). Fax: 314-447-8029. E-mail: journalscustomerservice-usa@elsevier.com (for print support); journalsonlinesupport-usa@elsevier. com (for online support).**

Reprints. For copies of 100 or more of articles in this publication, please contact the Commercial Reprints Department, Elsevier Inc., 360 Park Avenue South, New York, New York 10010-1710. Tel.: 212-633-3874; Fax: 212-633-3820; E-mail: reprints@elsevier.com.

Obstetrics and Gynecology Clinics of North America is also published in Spanish by McGraw-Hill Interamericana Editores S.A., P.O. Box 5-237, 06500, Mexico; in Portuguese by Reichmann and Affonso Editores, Rio de Janeiro, Brazil; and in Greek by Paschalidis Medical Publications, Athens, Greece.

Obstetrics and Gynecology Clinics of North America is covered in *MEDLINE/PubMed (Index Medicus), Excerpta Medica, Current Concepts/Clinical Medicine, Science Citation Index, BIOSIS, CINAHL,* and *ISI/BIOMED.*

Contributors

CONSULTING EDITOR

WILLIAM F. RAYBURN, MD, MBA
Distinguished Professor and Emeritus Chair, Department of Obstetrics and Gynecology, Associate Dean, Continuing Medical Education and Professional Development, University of New Mexico School of Medicine, Albuquerque, New Mexico

EDITORS

JANICE L. BACON, MD, FACOG
Women's Health and Diagnostic Center, Lexington Medical Center, West Columbia, South Carolina

PAUL G. TOMICH, MD
Professor, Department of Obstetrics and Gynecology, University of Nebraska Medical Center, Omaha, Nebraska

AUTHORS

JANICE L. BACON, MD, FACOG
Women's Health and Diagnostic Center, Lexington Medical Center, West Columbia, South Carolina

ASHA BHALWAL, MD
Division of Maternal-Fetal Medicine, Department of Obstetrics, Gynecology, and Reproductive Sciences, UT Health-University of Texas Medical School at Houston, Houston, Texas

CONSTANCE BOHON, MD, FACOG
Assistant Clinical Professor of Obstetrics and Gynecology, George Washington University School of Medicine and Health Sciences, Washington, DC

ELIZABETH R. BURTON, MD
Assistant Clinical Professor, Division of Gynecologic Oncology, Department of Obstetrics and Gynecology, Hanjani Institute of Gynecologic Oncology, Abington Hospital, Jefferson Health, The Sidney Kimmel Medical College, Thomas Jefferson University, Abington, Pennsylvania

LAURA M. CARLSON, MD
Clinical Fellow, Division of Maternal Fetal Medicine, Department of Obstetrics and Gynecology, University of North Carolina School of Medicine, Chapel Hill, North Carolina

SUNEET P. CHAUHAN, MD
Division of Maternal-Fetal Medicine, Department of Obstetrics, Gynecology, and Reproductive Sciences, UT Health-University of Texas Medical School at Houston, Houston, Texas

JOSHUA D. DAHLKE, MD
Division of Maternal-Fetal Medicine, Department of Obstetrics and Gynecology, Nebraska Methodist Women's Hospital and Perinatal Center, Omaha, Nebraska

DENISE M. ELSER, MD
Director, Urogynecology, Women's Health Institute of Illinois, Oak Lawn, Illinois

ANTHONY R. GREGG, MD, MBA, FACOG, FACMG
BL Stalnaker Professor, Director, Maternal Fetal Medicine, Department of Obstetrics and Gynecology, Director of Obstetrics, University of Florida Health System, University of Florida College of Medicine, Gainesville, Florida

JESSICA R. JACKSON, MD, MSBS
Adjunct Clinical Postdoctoral Fellow, Maternal Fetal Medicine, Department of Obstetrics and Gynecology, University of Florida College of Medicine, Gainesville, Florida

LYNN R. MACK, MD
Associate Professor, Division of Diabetes, Endocrinology & Metabolism, Department of Internal Medicine, The Nebraska Medical Center, Omaha, Nebraska

BENJIE BROWN MILLS, MD
Adjunct Professor of Pediatrics, Associate Professor, Department of Obstetrics & Gynecology, Greenville Health System, University of South Carolina School of Medicine–Greenville, Greenville, South Carolina

ROGER P. SMITH, MD
Assistant Dean for Graduate Medical Education, Professor of Clinical Biologic Sciences, Charles E. Schmidt College of Medicine, Florida Atlantic University, Boca Raton, Florida

JOEL I. SOROSKY, MD
Chair, Department of Obstetrics and Gynecology, Hanjani Institute of Gynecologic Oncology, Abington Hospital, Jefferson Health, The Sidney Kimmel Medical College, Thomas Jefferson University, Abington, Pennsylvania

PAUL G. TOMICH, MD
Professor, Department of Obstetrics and Gynecology, University of Nebraska Medical Center, Omaha, Nebraska

ERIN E. TRACY, MD, MPH
Associate Professor, Vincent Obstetrics and Gynecology, Obstetrics, Gynecology, and Reproductive Biology, Massachusetts General Hospital, Harvard Medical School, Boston, Massachusetts

NEETA L. VORA, MD
Assistant Professor, Division of Maternal Fetal Medicine, Department of Obstetrics and Gynecology, University of North Carolina School of Medicine, Chapel Hill, North Carolina

Contents

prevention with a focus on human papillomavirus vaccination and cervical cancer screening is reviewed, emphasizing the new focus of less frequent intervention in an effort to maintain high rates of early detection of disease while decreasing unnecessary and anxiety-provoking colposcopies, biopsies, and excisional procedures. The replacement of traditional endometrial hyperplasia terminology with more relevant clinical categories, with an emphasis on the introduction of endometrial intraepithelial neoplasia, is presented. Fertility-sparing options in the management of early cervical and endometrial cancers are reviewed.

Gestational diabetes mellitus (GDM) affects approximately 6% of pregnant women, and prevalence is increasing in parallel with the obesity epidemic. Protocols for screening/diagnosing GDM are controversial with several guidelines available. Treatment of GDM results in a reduction in the incidence of preeclampsia, shoulder dystocia, and macrosomia. If diet and lifestyle changes do not result in target glucose levels, then treatment with metformin, glyburide, or insulin should begin. It is generally recommended that pregnancies complicated by GDM do not go beyond term. For women identified to have prediabetes, intensive lifestyle intervention and metformin have been shown to prevent or delay progression to type 2 diabetes.

Systematic reviews with meta-analysis represent the highest level of evidence used to guide clinical practice. The defining criteria used to diagnose preeclampsia have evolved, and will likely continue to evolve. Proteinuria is sufficient but not necessary when defining preeclampsia. Hypertension without proteinuria but with severe features is diagnostic. The methods used to measure urinary protein have changed. The gold standard remains the 24-hour urine test. The efficacy of low-dose aspirin in preventing preeclampsia is a function of baseline risk. Data suggest that treating mild to moderate blood pressure has clear maternal benefits with little fetal or neonatal risk.

Shoulder dystocia and postpartum hemorrhage represent two of the most common emergencies faced in obstetric clinical practice, both requiring prompt recognition and management to avoid significant morbidity or mortality. Shoulder dystocia is an uncommon, unpredictable, and unpreventable obstetric emergency and can be managed with appropriate intervention. Postpartum hemorrhage occurs more commonly and carries significant risk of maternal morbidity. Institutional protocols and algorithms for the prevention and management of shoulder dystocia and postpartum hemorrhage have become mainstays for clinicians. The goal of this review is to summarize the diagnosis, incidence, risk factors, and management of shoulder dystocia and postpartum hemorrhage.

The American Congress of Obstetricians and Gynecologists recommends that all pregnant women be offered aneuploidy screening or diagnostic testing. A myriad of screening and testing options are available to patients based on their risk profile and gestational age. Screening options include traditional serum analyte screening, such as first-trimester screening or quadruple screening, and more recently, cell-free DNA. Diagnostic testing choices include chorionic villus sampling and amniocentesis. The number of screening and diagnostic modalities complicates prenatal counseling for physicians and can be difficult for patients to grasp. Appropriate pretest and posttest counseling is important to ensure adequate understanding of results and ensure testing strategy is concordant with patient goals.

Breast cancer is predicted to be the most common newly diagnosed cancer in women in 2016. Screening mammography is the most commonly used method for the detection of breast cancer in women of average risk. A genetic risk assessment is recommended for women with a greater than 20% to 25% chance of having a predisposition to breast and ovarian cancer. Evaluation of a breast mass begins with a detailed history, assessment for cancer risk, and physical examination.

Many women experience urogynecologic or pelvic floor disorders, especially urinary incontinence and pelvic organ prolapse. The obstetrician/gynecologist is often the first health care professional to evaluate and treat these disorders. Treatments include pelvic floor muscle training, behavioral therapies, oral medications, neuromodulation, intradetrusor medications, and surgery. When approaching the woman with symptomatic prolapse, familiarity with pessaries and various surgical procedures aid in counseling. Referral to a pelvic floor physical therapist or to a female pelvic medicine and reconstructive surgeon should be considered. Increasing attention to data on cost-effectiveness is a necessity.

A clear understanding of the physiology of the menopausal transition, clinical symptoms, and physical changes is essential for individualized patient management, maximizing benefits and minimizing risks for the present and the future. Menopause, defined by amenorrhea for 12 consecutive months, is determined retrospectively and represents a permanent end to menses. Many physical changes occur during the menopausal transition and beyond. Knowledge of symptoms and findings experienced by women undergoing the menopausal transition allow individualized care- improving quality of life and enhancing wellbeing for years to come.

Special Article

It is estimated that 40% to 75% of obstetricians and gynecologists currently suffer from professional burnout, making the lifetime risk a virtual certainty. Although these statistics make for a dismal view of the profession, if the causes and symptoms can be identified simple steps can be implemented to reverse the threat. With a little care, the enjoyment of practice can be restored and the sense of reward and the value of service can be returned.

OBSTETRICS AND GYNECOLOGY CLINICS

THE CLINICS ARE AVAILABLE ONLINE!
Access your subscription at:
www.theclinics.com

Foreword

Lifelong Learning Requires Maintenance of Knowledge

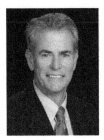

William F. Rayburn, MD, MBA
Consulting Editor

This issue of *Obstetrics and Gynecology Clinics of North America*, guest edited by Janice Bacon, MD and Paul Tomich, MD, deals with topics of clinical importance to the obstetrician-gynecologist for maintenance of knowledge. This issue resulted from a popular postgraduate course repeated at the American College of Obstetricians and Gynecologists Annual Clinical and Scientific Meeting. A portion of lecture material included topics presented in this issue: vaginitis beyond the basics, abnormal uterine bleeding, recognition of therapies for cervix and uterine malignancies, prenatal diagnostic screening, gestational diabetes, hypertension, peripartum obstetric emergencies, menopausal transition, common breast disorders, and recognizing and managing common urogynecologic disorders.

Maintenance of knowledge is critical for physician performance improvement and maintenance of certification (MOC). The goal of the MOC process, as prepared by the American Board of Obstetrics and Gynecology (ABOG), is to improve patient safety. This process helps to assure that Diplomates are maintaining a high level of current medical knowledge, and appropriately applying that information in their practices. Like this ABOG process, information reported in this issue was developed to enable physicians to maintain a high standard of current medical knowledge and safety.

In each year of a 6-year recertification cycle, Diplomates must complete a number of tasks, including reading current literature and answering questions about the content, and performing a quality improvement activity. In selected years, specific training in medical safety is included, and at the end of each cycle, a secure written examination must be passed. In addition, ABOG carefully reviews all adverse actions against physicians, as Diplomates are required to hold and maintain an unrestricted license to practice medicine.

Several past registrants have retaken this course due to its value in reconfirming and updating their knowledge about standard subjects, including cost containment and potential patient safety. This issue brings to the reader the most current knowledge

Obstet Gynecol Clin N Am 44 (2017) xi–xii
http://dx.doi.org/10.1016/j.ogc.2017.03.002
0889-8545/17/© 2017 Published by Elsevier Inc.

from the most recent course as presented and refined by the qualified lecturers. The authors have become more expert in their subject material and pass along their knowledge in this issue. We look forward to another update in the forthcoming years as part of lifelong learning.

William F. Rayburn, MD, MBA
Department of Obstetrics and Gynecology
University of New Mexico School of Medicine
MSC 10 5580, 1 University of New Mexico
Albuquerque, NM 87131-0001, USA

E-mail address:
WRayburn@salud.unm.edu

Preface

Maintenance of Knowledge

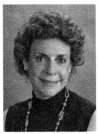 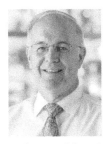

Janice L. Bacon, MD, FACOG   Paul G. Tomich, MD
Editors

Remaining current and up-to-date in today's rapidly expanding world of medical advances is challenging to all physicians. Providing efficient and appropriate clinical care, medical cost containment, and the potential to improve patient safety have also been aspects of continuing medical education endeavors.

In 2000, the US Medical Specialty Boards adopted Maintenance of Certification (MOC), a program incorporating education and assessment research and implementation as part of a quality-improvement framework recognizing physician performance as a crucial contributor to health outcomes. MOC focused on the core competencies of the American Board of Medical Specialties (ABMS) and the Accreditation Council for Graduate Medical Education, including professionalism, lifelong learning and self-assessment, cognitive expertise, and performance in practice.

The American Board of Obstetrics and Gynecology, a founding organization of the ABMS, developed a 6-year plan for maintenance of certification for obstetricians and gynecologists culminating in a standardized exam in year six.

To meet the needs of physicians desiring review and current information within the broad specialty of obstetrics and gynecology, the American College of Obstetrics and Gynecology began presenting Maintenance of Knowledge courses each year at their annual clinical meeting. Topics presented in the courses allowed physicians to receive current information in many areas of the specialty for review and preparation for the exam in year six. These courses also attracted physicians who simply wanted updates in a variety of topics and for residents or graduates preparing for their oral board exams.

This issue of *Obstetrics and Gynecology Clinics of North America* includes topics from the Maintenance of Knowledge courses with succinct information helpful to

Obstet Gynecol Clin N Am 44 (2017) xiii–xiv
http://dx.doi.org/10.1016/j.ogc.2017.03.001
0889-8545/17/© 2017 Published by Elsevier Inc.

obgyn.theclinics.com

students, residents, and clinicians. We are most appreciative to the authors who pre-pared these topics in this issue and hope they will be enjoyed by all readers.

Janice L. Bacon, MD, FACOG
Lexington Medical Park 1
2728 Sunset Boulevard
West Columbia, SC 29169, USA

Paul G. Tomich, MD
Division of Maternal Fetal Medicine
Department of Obstetrics and Gynecology
983255 Nebraska Medical Center
Omaha, NE 68198-3255, USA

E-mail addresses:
jlbacon@lexhealth.org (J.L. Bacon)
ptomich@unmc.edu (P.G. Tomich)

Contraception
Menarche to Menopause

Erin E. Tracy, MD, MPH

KEYWORDS

- Barrier methods • Hormonal contraception • Long-acting reversible contraception
- Sterilization • Intrauterine devices

KEY POINTS

- Unintended pregnancy rates remain unacceptably high, despite decades of research and advocacy.
- Newer literature supports the use of long-acting reversible contraception in most reproductive-aged women.
- Although there are more than 1800 recommendations regarding specific contraceptive tools in consideration of women's individual health statuses, most women have a wide selection of contraceptive options to safely consider.
- There are also several potential health benefits to contraception, including treatment of menorrhagia, dysmenorrhea, endometrial hyperplasia, malignancy chemoprophylaxis, and sexually transmitted disease prevention.

It is a widely touted fact that approximately 50% of pregnancies in the United States are unplanned.[1] Despite this statistical reality, that has been stable over decades, there has recently been a significant decrease in the rate of teen pregnancies (http://www.pewresearch.org/fact-tank/2016/04/29/why-is-the-teenbirth-rate-falling/).[2] A recent analysis by the Pew Research Center attributes this decrease to a multitude of factors, including economic challenges, decreased coital activity, better sex education, and the use of more effective contraception. Although contraception is nothing new, vigorous approaches to longer-acting methods have been quite effective. *Time Magazine* recently outlined the history of contraception.[3] Historical references include a 1550 BC Egyptian article entitled the *Ebers Papyrus* that discussed the construction of a vaginal pessary made out of dates, acacia, and honey as a paste and Casanova's memoirs approximately 2 centuries later that described sheep-bladder condoms and a half lemon used as a cervical cap. In Brooklyn in 1916 Margaret Sanger, a real pioneer in the field, opened the first family

Disclosure Statement: The author has nothing to disclose.
Vincent Obstetrics and Gynecology, Obstetrics, Gynecology, and Reproductive Biology, Massachusetts General Hospital, Harvard Medical School, Founders 406, 55 Fruit Street, Boston, MA 02114, USA
E-mail address: EETRACY@mgh.harvard.edu

Obstet Gynecol Clin N Am 44 (2017) 143–158
http://dx.doi.org/10.1016/j.ogc.2017.02.001
0889-8545/17/© 2017 Elsevier Inc. All rights reserved.

obgyn.theclinics.com

planning clinic in the United States, which was shut down in less than 2 weeks. Over time many laws were enacted prohibiting contraception, but in 1965 the US Supreme Court's *Griswold v Connecticut* ruling essentially overturned state laws banning contraception for married couples. Indeed the 1964 American Medical Association House of Delegates position stated that "an intelligent recognition of the problems that relate to human reproduction, including the need for population control, is more than a matter of responsible parenthood; it is a matter of responsible medical practice."[4] The US Food and Drug Administration (FDA) approved mestranol/norethynodrel, the first hormonal contraception, in May of 1960.[5] Despite significant advances in reproductive services since then, however, it is noteworthy that approximately 140 million around the world lack access to contraception.[6] In 2008, although 44% of maternal deaths (272,040 women) were prevented in 172 developing countries because of effective contraception, another 29% of maternal deaths could have been averted if there had been better contraceptive availability and practices.

TYPES OF CONTRACEPTION

There are a host of contraceptive choices, each with potential risks and benefits. These choices can be categorized according to mechanism, including natural family planning, barrier methods, hormonal systemic contraception, injectable progestins, long-acting reversible contraception (LARC), and permanent sterilization.

NATURAL FAMILY PLANNING

The US Department of Health and Human Services estimates that of 100 couples annually who use natural family planning up to 25 may become pregnant.[7] This method involves an analysis of a woman's menstrual cycle with particular emphasis on basal body temperature, cervical mucus, ovulation predictor kits, cycle beads, or the computation of cycle days. Barrier methods can be added to natural family planning techniques to improve efficacy. The barrier methods require personal skill regarding correct placement and insertion of the devices in addition to the commitment to regular consistent use.

BARRIER METHODS

Most barrier methods are used by female partners, including diaphragms, contraceptive sponges, cervical caps, and female condoms. Male partners' latex condoms can help decrease the risk of sexually transmitted diseases (STDs) in addition to a contraceptive benefit. Barrier methods have the added benefit of not being contraindicated for women with many systemic medical conditions that increase the risk of hormonal methods.

Diaphragms

Diaphragms require a prescription based on a clinician's appraisal of the appropriate size (size 60–90 mm) for a given patient (**Fig. 1**). The posterior rim of the device should sit comfortably in patients' posterior vaginal fornix, with the anterior rim tucked easily behind the pubic bone and the cervix should be palpable through its dome. It should be inserted before coitus and removed 6 hours later, 24 hours later at the latest. One of the advantages of diaphragms is women determine their timing and use. Although there are some studies indicating a decrease in STDs,

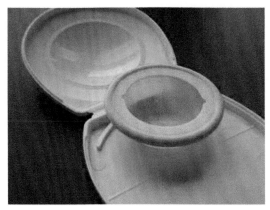

Fig. 1. Diaphragm. (*Courtesy of* CooperSurgical, Inc, Trumbull, CT; with permission.)

others report an increase in the risk of urinary tract infections and toxic shock syndrome.[8]

Contraceptive Sponges

The FDA has approved only a single type of sponge, the Today Sponge, for American markets[9] (**Fig. 2**). It must be inserted before coitus and has a strap to facilitate removal after intercourse. In addition to its polyurethane foam barrier mechanism, it also contains a spermicide. It must be washed with tap water before insertion, left in situ for 6 hours postcoitally, and used with each act of intercourse. Manufacturers cite an efficacy rate based on best practices of 84% to 87%.[10]

Cervical Caps

Like the sponge, there is only one type of cervical cap available in the United States, the FemCap silicone device (FemCap, Inc, Del Mar, CA).[11] Like the diaphragm, the cervical cap requires both a clinician's sizing the device and a prescription (**Fig. 3**). The 22-mm cap is generally for nulliparous patients, the 26-mm cap for someone who had a pregnancy of any duration, and the 30-mm cap for a parous woman who has had a vaginal delivery in the past. Failure rates range from 14% to

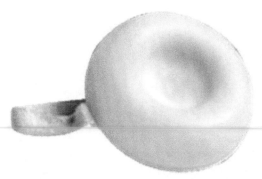

Fig. 2. The today sponge. (*Courtesy of* Mayer Laboratories, Inc, Sonoma, CA; with permission.)

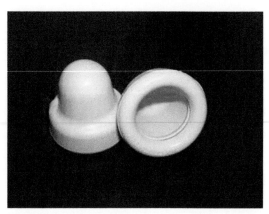

Fig. 3. Cervical caps.

29%.[12] It should be used with spermicide and left in the vagina for no fewer than 6 hours and no longer than 48 hours.

Female Condoms

Female condoms are either made of a strong plastic polyurethane or nitrile (**Fig. 4**). The ring of the condom is inserted into the vagina to cover the cervix, and the other end of the ring is open and sits outside of the vagina covering the vulva. Efficacy ranges from 75% to 92%.[13] They are available over the counter, so require neither a clinician's examination nor a prescription.

Male Condoms

Although male condoms require the cooperation of a male partner, they do have the added benefit of STD prevention. (Synthetic materials, such as latex, offer protection; older animal-derived devices do not.) They are for single use, must be used consistently, and should be kept in a cool dark place. Other specific tips include careful handling to avoid ripping the materials, placement after the penis becomes erect, avoidance of trapped air in the tip, and the use of water-based lubricants. (Oil-based lubricants could weaken the latex and increase the risk of breakage.)[14] Success rates approach 82%.[15]

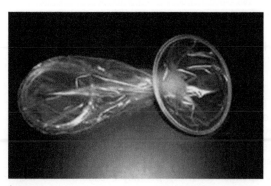

Fig. 4. Female condom.

Spermicide

Noxonyl-9 is the commercially available preparation either as a cream, film, gel, foam, or suppository. Spermicides should be used with both diaphragms and cervical caps. When used alone they should be placed at least 10 minutes before coitus. Although they immobilize sperm, they do not seem to protect against STDs.[16]

ORAL CONTRACEPTION

Oral contraceptive pills (OCPs) provide a myriad of benefits, including the treatment of abnormal uterine bleeding, hyperandrogenism (including polycystic ovarian syndrome) and dysmenorrhea, ovarian suppression (ie, for bleeding diatheses and cancer risk reduction), some medical benefits (ie, acne vulgaris), and the treatment of menstrual-related conditions, in addition to pregnancy prevention. Ethinyl estradiol (in most preparations) and a type of progestin are the active ingredients of combination OCPs. OCPs work by a variety of mechanisms, including the suppression of the hypothalamic pituitary axis (both gonadotropin-releasing hormone and pituitary gonadotropins), the inhibition of the midcycle luteinizing hormone surge and its resulting ovulation, and a decrease in the rate of the development of ovarian follicles. In addition to these effects by combination OCPs, the progestin component alters both the endometrial lining and cervical mucus resulting in less favorable conditions for implantation and fertilization.

Because of their systemic absorption and risk of potential deleterious side effects both the World Health Organization (WHO) and the Centers for Disease Control and Prevention (CDC) have developed a series of tables based on efficacy and preferred methods taking into consideration personal characteristics (ie, body mass index [BMI], smoking, age), past medical history (ie, malignancy, rheumatologic or cardiovascular diseases, history of thromboembolic events, hypertension, migraines with aura), and other potential risk factors (ie, thrombogenic mutations, renal or hepatic disease). In 2015 the WHO updated these guidelines.[17] Consideration of alternative methods is recommended for specific patient populations (ie, smokers older than 35 years, migraines with aura, cirrhosis, thromboembolic disease, cardiomyopathy, uncontrolled hypertension, cerebral vascular accidents, prolonged immobilization, and complicated vascular disease). There is a myriad of charts related to these classifications, which are best referenced directly at http://apps.who.int/iris/bitstream/10665/181468/1/9789241549158_eng.pdf. A summary of the CDC's recommendations is found in **Fig. 5.**[18] There is also an application (app) for this that can be downloaded to clinicians' personal devices for ease of reference. Consideration of decreased efficacy with the use of many anticonvulsants and with rifampin should steer one toward other methods of contraception in patients requiring these medications.[19]

Although most pills have doses of 30 to 35 mcg ethinyl estradiol, some preparations are 10 to 25 mcg. The lower dose preparations are sometimes used for perimenopausal women or patients leery of potential estrogen-related side effects; however, both breakthrough bleeding and amenorrhea are more common with the lower-dose regimens. There are several progestins used in combination pills. Many are derived from testosterone and, thus, bind both progesterone and androgen receptors, consequently having some androgenic risks (classified as both first- and second-generation progestins, including norethindrone and levonorgestrel). The third-generation progestins, such as norgestimate and desogestrel, have less androgenic affinity and, thus, less risk of adverse effects on lipids.[20] There is controversy, however, as to whether these new preparations increase the risk of thromboembolic

Condition	Sub-Condition	CHC	POP	Injection	Implant	LNG-IUD	Cu-IUD
		I / C	I / C	I / C	I / C	I / C	I / C
Age		Menarche to <40=1 ≥40=2	Menarche to <18=1 18-45=1 >45=1	Menarche to <18=2 18-45=1 >45=2	Menarche to <18=1 18-45=1 >45=1	Menarche to <20=2 ≥20=1	Menarche to <20=2 ≥20=1
Anatomic abnormalities	a) Distorted uterine cavity					4	4
	b) Other abnormalities					2	2
Anemias	a) Thalassemia	1	1	1	1	1	2
	b) Sickle cell disease‡	2	1	1	1	1	2
	c) Iron-deficiency anemia	1	1	1	1	1	2
Benign ovarian tumors	*(including cysts)*	1	1	1	1	1	1
Breast disease	a) Undiagnosed mass	2*	2*	2*	2*	2	1
	b) Benign breast disease	1	1	1	1	1	1
	c) Family history of cancer	1	1	1	1	1	1
	d) Breast cancer‡						
	i) current	4	4	4	4	4	1
	ii) past and no evidence of current disease for 5 years	3	3	3	3	3	1
Breastfeeding *(see also Postpartum)*	a) <1 month postpartum	3*	2*	2*	2*		
	b) 1 month or more postpartum	2*	1*	1*	1*		
Cervical cancer	Awaiting treatment	2	1	2	2	4 / 2	4 / 2
Cervical ectropion		1	1	1	1	1	1
Cervical intraepithelial neoplasia		2	1	2	2	2	1
Cirrhosis	a) Mild *(compensated)*	1	1	1	1	1	1
	b) Severe‡ *(decompensated)*	4	3	3	3	3	1
Deep venous thrombosis (DVT)/Pulmonary embolism (PE)	a) History of DVT/PE, not on anticoagulant therapy						
	i) higher risk for recurrent DVT/PE	4	2	2	2	2	1
	ii) lower risk for recurrent DVT/PE	3	2	2	2	2	1
	b) Acute DVT/PE	4	2	2	2	2	2
	c) DVT/PE and established on anticoagulant therapy for at least 3 months						
	i) higher risk for recurrent DVT/PE	4*	2	2	2	2	2
	ii) lower risk for recurrent DVT/PE	3*	2	2	2	2	2
	d) Family history *(first-degree relatives)*	2	1	1	1	1	1
	e) Major surgery						
	i) with prolonged immobilization	4	2	2	2	2	1
	ii) without prolonged immobilization	2	1	1	1	1	1
	f) Minor surgery without immobilization	1	1	1	1	1	1
Depressive disorders		1*	1*	1*	1*	1*	1*
Diabetes mellitus (DM)	a) History of gestational DM only	1	1	1	1	1	1
	b) Non-vascular disease						
	i) non-insulin dependent	2	2	2	2	2	1
	ii) insulin dependent‡	2	2	2	2	2	1
	c) Nephropathy/retinopathy/neuropathy‡	3/4*	2	3	2	2	1
	d) Other vascular disease or diabetes of >20 years' duration‡	3/4*	2	3	2	2	1

Condition	Sub-Condition	CHC	POP	Injection	Implant	LNG-IUD	Cu-IUD
		I / C	I / C	I / C	I / C	I / C	I / C
Endometrial cancer‡		1	1	1	1	4 / 2	4 / 2
Endometrial hyperplasia		1	1	1	1	1	1
Endometriosis		1	1	1	1	1	2
Epilepsy‡	*(see also Drug Interactions)*	1*	1*	1*	1*	1	1
Gallbladder disease	a) Symptomatic						
	i) treated by cholecystectomy	2	2	2	2	2	1
	ii) medically treated	3	2	2	2	2	1
	iii) current	3	2	2	2	2	1
	b) Asymptomatic	2	2	2	2	2	1
Gestational trophoblastic disease	a) Decreasing or undetectable ß-hCG levels	1	1	1	1	3	3
	b) Persistently elevated ß-hCG levels or malignant disease‡	1	1	1	1	4	4
Headaches	a) Non-migrainous	1* / 2*	1* / 1*	1* / 1*	1* / 1*	1* / 1*	1*
	b) Migraine						
	i) without aura, age <35	2* / 3*	1* / 2*	2* / 2*	2* / 2*	2* / 2*	1*
	ii) without aura, age ≥35	3* / 4*	1* / 2*	2* / 2*	2* / 2*	2* / 2*	1*
	iii) with aura, any age	4* / 4*	2* / 3*	2* / 3*	2* / 3*	2* / 3*	1*
History of bariatric surgery‡	a) Restrictive procedures	1	1	1	1	1	1
	b) Malabsorptive procedures	COCs: 3 P/R: 1	3	1	1	1	1
History of cholestasis	a) Pregnancy-related	2	1	1	1	1	1
	b) Past COC-related	3	2	2	2	2	1
History of high blood pressure during pregnancy		2	1	1	1	1	1
History of pelvic surgery		1	1	1	1	1	1
Human immunodeficiency virus (HIV)	High risk	1	1	1*	1	2 / 2	2 / 2
	HIV infected *(see also Drug Interactions)*‡	1*	1*	1*	1*	2 / 2	2 / 2
	AIDS *(see also Drug Interactions)*‡	1*	1*	1*	1*	3 / 2*	3 / 2*
	Clinically well on therapy	*If on treatment, see Drug Interactions*				2 / 2	2 / 2
Hyperlipidemias		2/3*	2*	2*	2*	2*	1*
Hypertension	a) Adequately controlled hypertension	3*	1*	2*	1*	1	1
	b) Elevated blood pressure levels *(properly taken measurements)*						
	i) systolic 140-159 or diastolic 90-99	3	1	2	1	1	1
	ii) systolic ≥160 or diastolic ≥100‡	4	2	3	2	2	1
	c) Vascular disease	4	2	3	2	2	1
Inflammatory bowel disease	*(Ulcerative colitis, Crohn's disease)*	2/3*	2	2	1	1	1

Fig. 5. A summary of the CDC's recommendations regarding contraceptive use. (1) No restriction (*method can be used*). (2) Advantages generally outweigh theoretic or proven risks. (3) Theoretic or proven risks usually outweigh the advantages. (4) Unacceptable health risk (*method not to be used*). C, continuation of contraceptive method; CHC, combined hormonal contraceptive (pill, patch, and ring); COC, combined oral contraceptive; CU-IUD, copper-containing intrauterine device; I, initiation of contraceptive method; LNG-IUD, levonorgestrel-releasing intrauterine device; NA, not applicable; P/R, patch/ring; POP, progestin-only pill. (*From* Centers for Disease Control and Prevention [CDC]. Summary chart of US medical eligibility criteria for contraceptive use. 2010. Available at: http://www.cdc.gov/reproductivehealth/unintendedpregnancy/pdf/legal_summary-chart_english_final_tag508.pdf. Accessed July 28, 2016.)

events.[21] Other newer progestins, such as drospirenone, have not only progestin-related effects but also antiandrogenic and antimineralocorticoid activity.[22] Thus, they may have a mild benefit related to weight and blood pressure. There are both monophasic and multiphasic dosing regimens, depending on either stable dosing or varying levels of hormones throughout the month. Patients either take their pills permitting monthly or other types of standard cycling or as continuous preparations. Contraceptive patches and rings have similar risk and side effect profiles as oral alternatives, although there is enhanced systemic estrogen absorption in the patch.

Progesterone-only contraceptive pills are excellent alternatives for women for whom combination pills are contraindicated (ie, patients with a history of thromboembolic events, significant vascular disease, or hypertension) or for newly postpartum patients initiating lactation.

EMERGENCY CONTRACEPTION

In 1974, the Yuzpe and colleagues'[23] regimen was published outlining the potential efficacy of a combination OCP regimen in the immediate postcoital period. There were significant side effects related to the high-dose estrogen administration, however. With time other oral regimens were adapted, including ulipristal and levonorgestrel. Two recent randomized controlled studies looking at the efficacy of these two medications revealed the risk of pregnancy was 3 times higher for obese women and 4 times higher for those who had intercourse the day before their estimated day of ovulation.[24] Consideration for patients in these situations should involve an intrauterine device (IUD) postcoital option. One trial involving almost 2000 reproductive-aged women who requested a postcoital IUD placement within 120 hours of intercourse resulted in zero pregnancies and a high continuation rate.[25] Although IUDs do not have the benefit of over-the-counter availability, like levonorgestrel, they should be considered in settings where practical.

INJECTABLE PROGESTIN

Depot medroxyprogesterone acetate (DMPA) can be administered both intramuscularly (150 mg/1 mL) and subcutaneously (104 mg/0.65 mL) every 13 weeks.[26] Although it is not considered an LARC method (which are defined as forgettable, not requiring readministration more than every 3 years),[27] it is of longer duration than the other methods previously described in this article. Progestin-only injectables typically involve regular interaction with a health care provider for administration but are excellent options for those for whom daily or regular compliance may be an issue. They can also be considered in patients for whom estrogen is contraindicated. It should not be a first-line agent, however, for a patient who is hoping to pursue pregnancy quickly after discontinuation of the method because of a potential for delayed response of fertility after therapy.[28] Depot Provera can be used for the treatment of menstrual disorders such as dysmenorrhea, and amenorrhea rates may approach 71%.[29] Patients should be aware of the risk of pregnancy of 6% with this method, however.[30]

LONG-ACTING REVERSIBLE CONTRACEPTION METHODS

The LARC methods include the IUD and progesterone implants. The American College of Obstetricians and Gynecologists has embarked on a campaign advocating the promotion of LARC among interested patients based on the high efficacy of these rates.[31] The increasing efficacy rates can be seen pictorially in **Fig. 6**.[32]

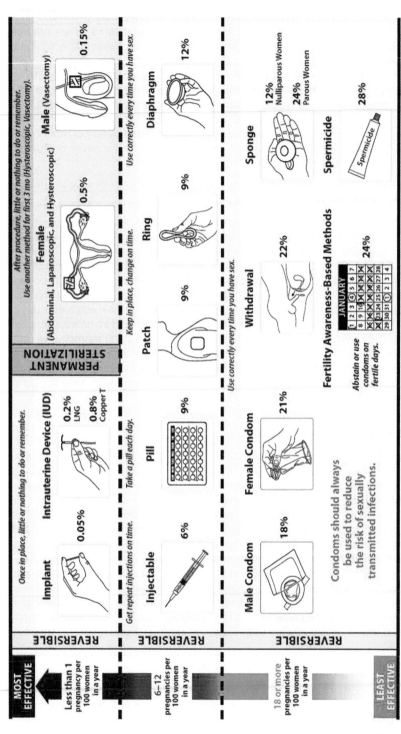

Fig. 6. Increasing efficacy rates of family planning methods. The percentages indicate the number out of every 100 women who experienced an unintended pregnancy within the first year of typical use of each contraceptive method. Other methods of contraception include the following: (1) Lactational amenorrhea method is a highly effective, temporary method of contraception. (2) Emergency contraception is emergency contraceptive pills or a

PROGESTERONE CONTRACEPTIVE IMPLANTS

The first polydimethylsiloxane (Silastic) tubes sealed with steroids came on the market in the early 1980s and used levonorgestrel, with a trade name of Norplant.[33] The initial 6-rod device was cumbersome in its removal and not as well tolerated as its eventual single-rod successor. The etonogestrel implant consists of a 40 mm × 2-mm semirigid plastic (ethylene vinyl acetate) rod containing 68 mg of the progestin etonogestrel (the 3-keto derivative of desogestrel), which is slowly released over at least 3 years.[34] Although the manufacturers initially studied the device in women of more ideal body weight, subsequent literature reveals comparable systemic levels of progestin across different BMIs.[35] The most recent 2016 US Medical Eligibility Criteria for Contraception lists this method as entirely compatible with obesity.[36] A multicenter trial of almost 1000 women revealed a pregnancy rate of less than 1%.[37] This study demonstrated a discontinuation rate of almost 15%, however, due to irregular bleeding. Short courses of combination OCPs and nonsteroidal antiinflammatory drugs may be beneficial in these settings. The safety profile of the progestin implant is noteworthy, however, because it can be used in women for whom estrogen is contraindicated. Its infrequent dosing is also potentially advantageous in consideration of both patient compliance and convenience. Unlike DMPA, the etonogestrel implant does not have an effect on bone density.[38] (The bone losses related to DMPA, however, are largely reversible after discontinuation of that method.[39]) It may also be an effective therapy for dysmenorrhea.[40]

INTRAUTERINE DEVICES

Most women are potential candidates for IUD therapy. There are few absolute contraindications, including recent puerperal sepsis and immediately after septic abortion.[41] There are 2 types of commercially available IUDs, including the copper IUD (Cu-T-380A) and the levonorgestrel IUD. The former is a T-shaped plastic device with 380 mm of copper wire encircling the stem and arms, with an FDA-approved duration for up to 10 years of use. The latter is also T shaped, consisting of a polyethylene frame containing 52 mg of levonorgestrel, with 20 μg released daily, which is approved for up to 5 years of use.[42] In 2013 the FDA approved a newer progestin IUD, with the trade name of Skyla, which has a slightly smaller diameter and is approved for up to 3 years of continuous use.[43] This last device is sometimes chosen preferentially for nulliparous patients, although parity is not a contraindication for any type of IUD.

Although more than 160 million women currently use IUDs, the story of IUDs is laced with controversy. They were first introduced in the early 1900s, but the Dalkron Shield's negative press and litigation (associated with sepsis and perforations, culminating in a $2.5 billion settlement in 1989) resulted in a significant decrease in their use.[44]

◄───

copper IUD after unprotected intercourse that substantially reduces risk of pregnancy. (*Adapted from* World Health Organization [WHO] Department of Reproductive Health and Research, Johns Hopkins Bloomberg School of Public Health/Center for Communication Programs [CCP]. Knowledge for health project. Family planning: a global handbook for providers [2011 update]. Baltimore [MD]; Geneva [Switzerland]: CCP; WHO; 2011; and Trussell J. Contraceptive failure in the United States. Contraception 2011;83:397–404; and *From* Centers for Disease Control and Prevention [CDC]. Effectiveness of Family Planning Methods. Available at: https://www.cdc.gov/reproductivehealth/unintendedpregnancy/pdf/family-planning-methods-2014.pdf. Accessed August 5, 2016.)

The copper IUD has a failure rate of less than 1%, with the most common side effects being irregular bleeding and pain.[45] IUDs make the cervix and the endometrium less favorable for the migration of both ova and sperm and for embryo implantation. All IUDs have a low risk of both expulsion and uterine perforation, but patients should be counseled about the potential for both. Both IUDs and progestin implants may be used in the immediate postpartum period, although expulsion rates for the former are higher than in the nonobstetrical population.[46] The copper IUD has the additional benefit of potentially being used for patients for whom hormonal therapy is contraindicated (ie, active breast cancer.) Levonorgestrel IUDs can be used for the treatment of endometrial hyperplasia, dysmenorrhea, menorrhagia and irregular bleeding. Indeed a recent meta-analysis suggests approximately half of women who may otherwise need a hysterectomy for menstrual regulation can avoid surgery using these devices.[47] Although IUDs are foreign objects, neither routine antibiotic administration nor cervical cultures are necessary before insertion, according to the 2011 guidelines form the American Congress of Obstetricians and Gynecologists (ACOG).[48] Although the incidence of pregnancy is decreased with the utilization of IUDs, if a patient were to become pregnant, her risk of ectopic pregnancy would be higher than women with otherwise spontaneous pregnancies. The location of the pregnancy must be identified; consequently, women for whom an intrauterine pregnancy is identified should have their IUDs removed because of the risk of both miscarriage and infection.

STERILIZATION

According to 2010 data in the United States of women using some form of contraception, 27% have had a tubal ligation and 10% rely on their partners having had vasectomies.[49] Vasectomies are usually done with local anesthetic, as an office procedure, and have a very low rate of complications (including infection and hematoma.) Vasectomies are the most cost-effective, safest permanent method of sterilization with similar efficacy rates as procedures in female counterparts.

A recent analysis of the Collaborative Review of Sterilization (CREST) study revealed women who have permanent sterilization do not have any change in sexual functioning.[50] There is a significant risk of ectopic pregnancy, however, with one-third of pregnancies in that setting being extrauterine.[51]

Bilateral tubal ligation can be done in the postpartum setting (as a separate procedure or during an abdominal delivery) or in the gynecologic population. Tubal ligations were first proposed as a technique in 1823 and remained an abdominal technique until the approval of Essure, a hysteroscopic approach, by the FDA in 2002.[52] Over the years different laparoscopic approaches were developed, including the use of cauterization, fallope rings (Band Disposable Kits by Circon/Gyrus ACMI, Fort Lauderdale, FL), Filshie clips (CooperSurgical, Trumbull, CT), and Hulka clips (Richard Wolf Medical Instruments Corp., Vernon Hills, IL). Current hysteroscopic tubal ligation guidelines necessitate both 3 months of postprocedural contraception and a confirmatory hysterosalpingogram. Comparative analyses reveal similar risks and benefits of the laparoscopic and hysteroscopic procedures.[53] The hysteroscopic approach has the potential benefit of decreased risk of injury to intra-abdominal structures, decreased pain, more rapid recovery, and potential availability as an office procedure with local analgesia. Any patient considering a permanent procedure should be counseled regarding the risk of regret and the availability of other reversible methods of high efficacy, such as LARC. Unfortunately, the prevalence of women who have had permanent sterilization procedures who subsequently regret that decision can be as high as 2% to 30%.[54]

SPECIFIC POPULATION CONSIDERATIONS

There is good evidence pregnancy spacing improves outcomes for subsequent pregnancies.[55] Providers can consider postpartum administration of LARC methods to improve both compliance and access. Estrogen-containing methods are potentially more risky, however, in light of the known thromboembolic risk in the postpartum period that can be as much as 5 times higher than during the antepartum period.[56] The lactational amenorrhea method (requiring all of the following 3 criteria: exclusive breastfeeding, amenorrhea, and less than 6 months postpartum) can provide contraception rates of 98%, although some studies report 25% rates in regular use.[57]

Teen pregnancy rates are reviewed earlier in this article. The United States continues to have one of the highest teen pregnancy rates of all industrialized countries.[58] The large prospective cohort Contraceptive CHOICE project revealed that women younger than 21 years who used short-acting contraception were almost twice as likely to have unintended pregnancies than their older counterparts.[59] Thus, LARC is potentially especially beneficial in this population. Condoms should be recommended as well for their role in the prevention of sexually transmitted infections.

Obese patients may potentially benefit from hormonal methods, and they should be counseled regarding recent Cochrane reviews that revealed no relationship between combination OCPs or the patch on weight gain and limited evidence of weight gain in 5 of the 16 progestin-only studies.[60]

Although women older than 40 years have declining fertility, they are still at risk for unintended pregnancies. There are no contraceptive methods that are contraindicated based on age alone, although patients should be evaluated for other potential medical comorbidities in contraceptive counseling.[61]

There is a myriad of health conditions that should be considered in the selection of the appropriate contraception for an individual patient, based on her individual risk status. Indeed the WHO's "Medical Eligibility Criteria for Contraceptive Use" includes more than 1800 recommendations for more than 120 medical conditions.[62] In evaluating the risks and benefits of contraception in potentially high-risk patients, however, it is important to also review the risks pregnancy would pose to them were they to become gravid.

POLICY IMPLICATIONS

In recognition of the steady unacceptably high rates of unintended pregnancy in the United States and the importance of removing barriers to access and care, in 2015 the ACOG advocated for "over-the-counter access to oral contraceptives with accompanying full insurance coverage or cost supports."[63] This support was partly in response to studies revealing increased compliance removing the prescription requirement.[64]

In a similar vein, in August of 2016 the ACOG's Committee on Obstetric Practice advocated for immediate postpartum LARC as potentially efficacious for postpartum women with few medical contraindications.[65] The ACOG has had a similar advocacy effort supporting increased use of contraceptive implants and IUDs for sexually active women, including nulliparous and adolescent patients.[66] The ACOG has also actively promoted providers' use of the "US Medical Eligibility Criteria for Contraceptive Use," issued by the CDC.[67]

TOOLS FOR PROVIDERS

Bedsider.org has a wealth of information about contraception for both patients and providers.[68] It also has tools to improve compliance with birth control and appointment reminders and information about available providers. Practices can use its patient education materials as well.

The CDC has an iPhone/iPad app that was recently updated based on the "US Medical Eligibility Criteria for Contraceptive Use, 2016," which gives providers an interactive tool to access the greater than 1800 recommendations to be considered when selecting appropriate methods for patients.[69]

The ACOG LARC program also maintains a frequently updated list of resources for both providers and patients at http://www.acog.org/About-ACOG/ACOG-Departments/Long-Acting-Reversible-Contraception/LARC-Practice-Resources.[70]

REFERENCES

1. Centers for Disease Control and Prevention. Unintended pregnancy prevention. Available at: https://www.cdc.gov/reproductivehealth/unintendedpregnancy/. Accessed July 26, 2016.
2. Patten E, Livingston G. Why is the teen birth rate falling?. Available at: http://www.pewresearch.org/fact-tank/2016/04/29/why-is-the-teen-birth-rate-falling/. Accessed July 26, 2016.
3. Time: A brief history of birth control. 2010. Available at: http://content.time.com/time/printout/0, 8816, 1983970,00.html#. Accessed July 26, 2016.
4. Reiling J. JAMA revisited: birth control in comprehensive health car. JAMA 2014; 312:194.
5. Christin-Maitre S. History of oral contraceptive drugs and their use worldwide. Best Pract Res Clin Endocrinol Metab 2013;27:3–12.
6. Espey E. Feminism and the moral imperative for contraception. Obstet Gynecol 2015;126:396–400.
7. U.S. Department of Health & Human Services. Fertility awareness (Natural family planning): The Facts. Available at: http://www.hhs.gov/opa/reproductive-health/contraception/natural-family-planning/index.html. Accessed July 28, 2016.
8. Allen R. Diaphragm fitting. Fam Physician 2004;69:97–100.
9. May Clinic. Contraceptive sponge. Available at: http://www.mayoclinic.org/tests-procedures/contraceptive-sponge/home/ovc-20166778?p=1. Accessed July 28, 2016.
10. Available at: http://todaysponge.com/effectiveness.html. Accessed July 28, 2016.
11. Association of Reproductive Health Professionals. Choosing a birth control method: Cervical Cap. Available at: http://www.arhp.org/publications-and-resources/quick-reference-guide-for-clinicians/choosing/cervical-cap. Accessed July 28, 2016.
12. U.S Food and Drug Administration. FemCap-P020041. Available at: http://www.fda.gov/MedicalDevices/ProductsandMedicalProcedures/DeviceApprovalsandClearances/Recently-ApprovedDevices/ucm082597.htm. Accessed July 28, 2016.
13. National Institutes of Health/U.S. National Library of Medicine: Medine Plus. Female condoms. Available at: https://medlineplus.gov/ency/article/004002.htm. Accessed July 28, 2016.
14. Center for disease control and prevention (CDC). Update: barrier protection against HIV infection and other sexually transmitted diseases. MMWR Morb Mortal Wkly Rep 1993;42:589–91.
15. Association of Reproductive Health Professionals. Choosing a birth control method: Male condoms. Available at: http://www.arhp.org/Publications-and-Resources/

Quick-Reference-Guide-for-Clinicians/choosing/Male-condom. Accessed July 28, 2016.

16. Kreiss J, Ngugi E, Holmes K, et al. Efficacy of nonoxynol 9 contraceptive sponge use in prevention heterosexual acquisition of HIV in Nairobi prostitutes. JAMA 1992;268:477.

17. World Health Organization. 5th edition Medical eligibility criteria for contraceptive use. Geneva (Switzerland): World Health Organization; 2015. Available at: http://apps.who.int/iris/bitstream/10665/181468/1/9789241549158_eng.pdf. Accessed July 28, 2016.

18. Center for Disease Control. Summary chart of U.S. medical eligibility criteria for contraceptive use. 2010. Available at: http://www.cdc.gov/reproductivehealth/unintendedpregnancy/pdf/legal_summary-chart_english_final_tag508.pdf. Accessed July 28, 2016.

19. Barditch-Crove P, Trapnell C, Ette E, et al. The effects of rifampin and rifabutin on the pharmacokinetics and pharmacodynamics of a combination oral contraceptive. Clin Pharmacol Ther 1999;65:428.

20. Phillips A, Hahn D, McGuire J. Preclinical evaluation of norgestimate, a progestin with minimal androgenic activity. Am J Obstet Gynecol 1992;167:1191.

21. Vandenbroucke J, Rosendasl F. End of the line for "third-generation-pill" controversy? Lancet 1997;349:1113–4.

22. Foldart J, Wutke W, Bouw G, et al. A comparative investigation of contraceptive reliability, cycle control and tolerance of two monophasic oral contraceptives containing either drospirenone or desogestrel. Eur J Contracept Reprod Health Care 2000;5:124.

23. Yuzpe A, Thurlow H, Ramzy I, et al. Post coital contraception-A pilot study. J Reprod Med 1974;13:53–6.

24. Glasier A, Cameron S, Blithe D, et al. Can we identify women at risk of pregnancy despite using emergency contraception? Data from randomized trials of ulipristal acetate and levonorgestrel. Contraception 2011;84:363.

25. Wu S, Godfrey E, Wojdyla D, et al. Copper T380A intrauterine device for emergency contraception: a prospective, multicentre, cohort clinical trial. BJOG 2010;117:1205.

26. Kaunitz A. Depot medroxyprogesterone acetate for contraception. Up to Date, Netherlands: Wolters Kluwer; 2016. Available at: https://www.uptodate.com/contents/depot-medroxyprogesterone-acetate-for-contraception?topicKey=OBGYN%2F5468&elapsedTimeMs=16&source=search_result&searchTerm=depo+provera&selectedTitle=2%7E43&view=print&displayedView=full#. Accessed August 2, 2016.

27. Grimes D. Forgettable contraception. Contraception 2009;30:497–9.

28. Schwallie P, Assenzo J. The effect of depot medroxyprogesterone acetate on pituitary and ovarian function, and the return of fertility following its discontinuation: a review. Contraception 1974;10:181–202.

29. Arias R, Jain J, Brucker C, et al. Changes in bleeding patterns with depot medroxyprogesterone acetate subcutaneous injection 104 mg. Contraception 2006;74:234–8.

30. Trussell J. Contraceptive failure in the United States. Contraception 2011;83:397.

31. American College of Obstetricians and Gynecologists. Long-acting reversible contraception program. Available at: http://www.acog.org/About-ACOG/ACOG-Departments/Long-Acting-Reversible-Contraception. Accessed August 2, 2016.

32. Centers for Disease Control and Prevention. Available at: https://www.cdc.gov/reproductivehealth/unintendedpregnancy/pdf/family-planning-methods-2014.pdf. Accessed August 5, 2016.

33. Associate of Reproductive Health Professionals. The single-rod contraceptive implant. Available at: http://www.arhp.org/publications-and-resources/clinical-proceedings/Single-Rod/History. Accessed August 2, 2016.

34. Darney P. Etonogestrel contraceptive implant. UpToDate; 2016. Available at: http://www.uptodate.com/contents/etonogestrel-contraceptive-implant?topicKey=OBGYN%2F3266&elapsedTimeMs=14&source=search_result&searchTerm=nexplanon&selectedTitle=4%7E41&view=print&displayedView=full#. Accessed August 2, 2016.

35. Morrell K, Cremers S, Westhoff C, et al. Relationship between etonogestrel level and BMI in women using the contraceptive implant for more than 1 year. Contraception 2016;93:263.

36. Curtis KM, Tepper NK, Jatlaoui TC, et al. U.S. Medical Eligibility Criteria for Contraceptive Use, 2016. MMWR Recomm Rep 2016;65(3):1–104.

37. Darney P, Patel A, Rosen K, et al. Safety and efficacy of a single-rod etonogestrel implant (Implanon): results from 11 international clinical trials. Fertil Steril 2009;91:1646.

38. Sarfati S, deVemejoul M. Impact of combined and progesterone-only contraceptive on bone mineral density. Joint Bone Spine 2009;76:134–8.

39. Berenson A, Rahman M, Breitkopf C, et al. Effects of depot medroxyprogesterone acetate and the 20-microgram oral contraceptives on bone mineral density. Obstet Gynecol 2008;112:788–99.

40. Funk S, Miller M, Mishell D, et al. Safety and efficacy of Implanon, a single rod implantable contraceptive containing etonogestrel. Contraception 2005;71:319–26.

41. American College of Obstetricians and Gynecologists Committee Opinion. Adolescents and long-acting reversible contraception: implants and intrauterine devices. 2012;539:1–7.

42. Espey E, Ogburn T. Long-acting reversible contraceptives: intrauterine devices and the contraceptive implant. Obstet Gynecol 2011;117:705–19.

43. Department of Health and Human Services, Food and Drug Administration. Pediatric postmarketing pharmacovigilance and drug utilization review. 2016. Available at: http://www.fda.gov/downloads/AdvisoryCommittees/CommitteesMeetingMaterials/PediatricAdvisoryCommittee/UCM494490.pd,n. Accessed August 2, 2016.

44. Case Western Reserve University. History of contraception-IUD. Available at: http://www.case.edu/affil/skuyhistcontraception/online-2012/IUDs.html. Accessed August 2, 2016.

45. Brockmeyer A, Kishen M, Webb A. Experience of IUD/IUS insertions and clinical performance in nulliparous woman-a pilot study. Eur J Contracept Reprod Health Care 2008;13:248–54.

46. Dahlke J, Terpstra E, Ramseyer A, et al. Postpartum insertion of levonorgestrel-intrauterine system at three time periods: a prospective randomized pilot study. Contraception 2011;84:244–8.

47. Hurskainen R, Teperi J, Rissanen P, et al. Clinically outcomes and costs with the levonorgesterel-releasing intrauterine system or hysterectomy for treatment of menorrhagia: randomized trial 5- year follow up. JAMA 2004;291:1456–63.

48. American College of Obstetricians and Gynecologists. Long-acting reversible contraception: implants and intrauterine devices. Obstet Gynecol 2011;1212:1–13.
49. Jones J, Daniels K. Current contraceptive use in the United States, 2006-2010. And changes in patterns of use since 1995, vol. 60. Hyattsville (MD): National Health Statistics Reports; 2012.
50. Shih G, Zhang V, Bukowski K, et al. Bringing men to the table: sterilization can be for him or her. Clin Obstet Gynecol 2014;57:731–40.
51. Peterson H, Xia Z, Hughes J, et al. The risk of ectopic pregnancy after tubal sterilization. US collaborative review of sterilization working group. N Engl J Med 1997;336:762–7.
52. Zurawin R, Rivlin M. Tubal sterilization: History of the procedure. Available at: http://emedicine.medscape.com/article/266799-overview#a6. Accessed August 2, 2016.
53. Ouzounelli M, Reaven N. Essure hysteroscopic sterilization versus interval laparoscopic bilateral tubal ligation: a comparative effectiveness review. J Minim Invasive Gynecol 2015;22:342–52.
54. Hirshfeld-Cytron J, Winter J. Laparoscopic tubal renastomosis versus in vitro fertilization: cost-based decision analysis. Am J Obstet Gynecol 2013;209:56e1–6.
55. Kennedy K, Rivera R, McNeilly A. Consensus statement on the use of breastfeeding as a family planning method. Contraception 1989;39:477–96.
56. Heit J, Kobbervig C, James E, et al. Trends in the incidence of venous thromboembolism during pregnancy or postpartum: a 30 year population-based study. Ann Intern Med 2005;143:697–706.
57. Sober S, Schreiber C. Postpartum contraception. Clin Obstet Gynecol 2014;4:763–76.
58. Truehart A, Whitaker A. Contraception and the adolescent patient. Obstet Gynecol Surv 2015;70:263–73.
59. Winner B, Peipert J, Zhao Q, et al. Effectiveness of long-acting reversible contraception. N Engl J Med 2012;366:1998–2007.
60. Mody S, Han M. Obesity and contraception. Clin Obstet Gynecol 2014;57:501–7.
61. Allen R, Cwiak C, Kaunitz A. Contraception in women over 40 years of age. CMAJ 2013;185:565–73.
62. Lathrop E, Jatlaoiu T. Contraception for women with chronic medical conditions: an evidence-based approach. Clin Obstet Gynecol 2014;57:674–81.
63. American College of Obstetricians and Gynecologists. Access to contraception. Obstet Gynecol 2015;125:250–5.
64. Potter J, McKinnon S, Hopkins K, et al. Continuation of prescribed compared with over-the-counter oral contraceptives. Obstet Gynecol 2011;117:551–7.
65. American College of Obstetricians and Gynecologists. Immediate postpartum long-acting reversible contraception. 2016. Available at: http://www.acog.org/Resources-And-Publications/Committee-Opinions/Committee-on-Obstetric-Practice/Immediate-Postpartum-Long-Acting-Reversible-Contraception. Accessed August 4, 2016.
66. American College of Obstetricians and Gynecologists. Increasing access to contraceptive implants and intrauterine devices to reduce unintended pregnancy. 2015. Available at: http://www.acog.org/Resources-And-Publications/Committee-Opinions/Committee-on-Gynecologic-Practice/Increasing-Access-to-Contraceptive-Implants-and-Intrauterine-Devices-to-Reduce-Unintended-Pregnancy. Accessed August 4, 2016.
67. American College of Obstetricians and Gynecologists. Understanding and using the U.S. medical eligibility criteria for contraceptive use, 2010. 2011. Available at:

http://www.acog.org/Resources-And-Publications/Committee-Opinions/Committee-on-Gynecologic-Practice/Understanding-and-Using-the-US-Medical-Eligibility-Criteria-for-Contraceptive-Use-2010. Accessed August 4, 2016.
68. Available at: https://bedsider.org. Accessed August 4, 2016.
69. Available at: https://itunes.apple.com/WebObjects/MZStore.woa/wa/viewSoftware?id=595752188&mt=8. Accessed August 4, 2016.
70. Available at: http://www.acog.org/About-ACOG/ACOG-Departments/Long-Acting-Reversible-Contraception/LARC-Practice-Resources. Accessed August 4, 2016.

Vaginitis: Beyond the Basics

Benjie Brown Mills, MD

KEYWORDS

- Vaginitis • Vulvovaginal candidiasis • Candida • Bacterial vaginosis
- Trichomoniasis • Desquamative inflammatory vaginitis • Atrophic vaginitis

KEY POINTS

- Vaginal complaints such as discharge, odor, irritation, and itching are a very common reason women seek the help of a health care provider.
- Most patients are correctly diagnosed and treated, but some go on to have no resolution of symptoms with treatment or rapidly recurring symptoms.
- Vulvovaginal candidiasis, bacterial vaginosis, and trichomoniasis are the most common vaginitides. Uncomplicated cases are easy to treat and have very successful outcomes.
- Patients with chronic or recurrent vaginal complaints need an accurate diagnosis and other, rarer, conditions need to be ruled out.
- Once the correct diagnosis is made, effective therapeutic options for cure and symptom control can be implemented.

BACKGROUND

Vaginal symptoms are one of the most common reasons women seek care with a health care provider.[1] Women can experience a decrease in their quality of life from discomfort and pain, absence from work or school, disturbance in sexual function, anxiety, and a change in their self-image. After treatment, most of these symptoms resolve without any further issues, but some women do not get better with therapy, recur frequently, or never receive a correct diagnosis after initial therapy fails.[2]

The term "vaginitis" is a general diagnosis that includes a wide array of conditions in every age group. Of these, uncomplicated bacterial vaginosis (BV), vulvovaginal candidiasis, and trichomoniasis are diagnosed in 70% of patients.[3] Of those, 40% to 50% have BV, 20% to 25% have vaginal candidiasis, and 15% to 20% have trichomoniasis.[4] The remaining 30% are undiagnosed and, among others, can have physiologic discharge (leukorrhea), atrophic vaginitis, vulvar dermatologic abnormalities, or vulvodynia.[3,5]

Although uncomplicated, acute, single episodes of vaginitis may be quite simple to diagnose and treat, women with recurrent or continuous symptoms may have

Disclosure: The author has nothing to disclose.
Department of Obstetrics & Gynecology, Greenville Health System, University of South Carolina School of Medicine–Greenville, 890 West Faris Road, Suite 470, Greenville, SC 29605, USA
E-mail address: bmills@ghs.org

Obstet Gynecol Clin N Am 44 (2017) 159–177
http://dx.doi.org/10.1016/j.ogc.2017.02.010
obgyn.theclinics.com

seen many different health care providers with multiple attempted therapeutic agents.[2] Patients are often frustrated and present a therapeutic challenge for health care providers. Given the decrease in quality of life created by these symptoms, a methodical evaluation with consideration of a broad differential diagnosis is necessary.[2]

Diagnoses (other than the common vaginitides) that present as vaginal complaints include physiologic discharge, desquamative inflammatory vaginitis (DIV), cytolytic vaginosis, chronic vulvar diseases, atrophic vaginitis, localized provoked vestibulodynia, contact dermatitis, erosive lichen planus, or other unusual conditions. Multiple diagnoses can quickly complicate evaluation and management.[2,6] Thus, the art of history taking and physical examination is a must for appropriate diagnosis; however, clinical evaluation alone has been shown to be insufficient for the diagnosis of vaginitis.[2,7]

THE VAGINAL ECOSYSTEM

A delicate equilibrium, the vaginal ecosystem consists of a variety of bacteria and metabolic products from the microbes and the host. Acids, carbohydrates, proteins, and nucleic acids, fatty acids, and sugars from degrading bacteria are present.[8] There are nonpathogenic and pathogenic microbial species that exist in a ratio of approximately 200:1 (**Table 1**).[8] Under the right conditions, nonpathogenic bacteria can cause

Table 1
Nonpathogenic and pathogenic bacteria found endogenously in a healthy vaginal ecosystem

Facultative Anaerobic Bacteria		
Gram Positive	**Gram Negative**	**Gram Variable**
Lactobacillus crispatus	Escherichia coli[a]	Gardnerella spp.[a]
Lactobacillus casei	Enterobacter agglomerans[a]	
Lactobacillus gasseris	Enterobacter aerogenes[a]	
Lactobacillus insers	Enterobacter cloacae[a]	
Lactobacillus jensei	Klebsiella oxytoca	
Nonhemolytic streptococci	Klebsiella pneumonia	
Streptococcus agalactiae[a]	Morganella morganii[a]	
Streptococcus viridans	Proteus mirabilis	
Staphylococcus epidermidis	Proteus vulgaris	
Enterococcus faecalis[a]	Mycoplasma spp.[a]	
	Ureaplasma spp.[a]	
	Haemophilus influenzae[a]	

Obligate Anaerobic Bacteria	
Gram Positive	**Gram Negative**
Eubacterium spp.	Fusobacterium necrophorum[a]
Peptococcus niger[a]	Fusobacterium nucleatum[a]
Peptostreptococcus anaerobius[a]	Prevotella bivia[a]
Corynebacterium spp.	Prevotella melaninogenica[a]
	Veillonella spp.
	Mobiluncus spp.[a]

[a] Pathogenic organism.

Adapted from Faro S. Healthy vaginal ecosystem. In: Vaginitis: differential diagnosis and management. New York: The Parthenon Publishing Group; 2004. p. 13–20; and Workowski KA, Bolan GA. Centers for Disease Control and Prevention. Sexually transmitted diseases treatment guidelines, 2015. MMWR Recomm Rep 2015;64(No. RR–3):69–77.

symptoms. Disruption or imbalance of the ecosystem results in dominance of nonpathogenic and pathogenic bacteria over *Lactobacillus* and increases risk for BV or bacterial vaginitis.[9] It can be difficult to determine the cause of infection because Gram-positive and -negative, as well as aerobic and anaerobic bacteria can be found in a healthy vagina.[9] Pathogenic bacteria such as *Pseudomonas* spp., *Staphylococcus aureus*, *Escherichia coli*, *Enterobacter* spp., and *Haemophilus influenzae* have been isolated from asymptomatic, healthy women.[9] Colonization with pathogenic bacteria has been associated with adverse outcomes of pregnancy, such as chorioamnionitis and endometritis.[9] Infectious complications from gynecologic procedures are more likely if the vaginal ecosystem is disrupted, so much so that screening patients preoperatively for abnormalities on wet preparation has been suggested.[9]

Specific *Lactobacillus* species are responsible for maintaining the healthy vagina (see **Table 1**).[9] Typically only 1 species exists, which inhibits pathogenic bacteria in 3 ways[10,11]:

1. Production of organic acids (specifically lactic acid), which maintains a pH between 3.8 and 4.2,
2. Secretion of hydrogen peroxide, and
3. Lactocin production.

Not all *Lactobacillus* species can perform this duty if they cannot secrete significant amounts of the required elements.[12] Although *Lactobacillus* grows best in a pH greater than 4.5, it can grow in a lower pH between 3.8 and 4.5, whereas other bacterial inhabitants of the vagina either do not grow at a pH below 4.0, or grow poorly at a pH of 4.0 to 4.5.[13]

The Role of Estrogen

The lack of estrogen in the prepubertal and postmenopausal states results in a thin vaginal epithelium with a high pH ($\geq$4.7). The ecosystem before puberty contains a different variety of organisms from that which is fully estrogenized, and includes skin and fecal flora.[2] Colonization of *Lactobacilli* is encouraged by estrogen stimulation of glycogen with subsequent decrease in pH to less than 4.7.[5] Addition of estrogen causes an increase in vaginal discharge, which often leads to the conclusion that the patient has vulvovaginal candidiasis, despite objective evidence on physical examination and office-based laboratory testing to the contrary. This misinterpretation can result in inappropriate diagnosis and treatment.[2] In the postmenopausal patient, atrophic vaginitis may be the cause of discharge, particularly in the setting of vaginal dryness, dyspareunia, and irritation.

EVALUATION OF VAGINAL COMPLAINTS
History and Physical Examination

History and physical examination are vital to the proper diagnosis of vaginal symptoms. Patient history should include the characteristics of the discharge such as color, consistency, and amount.[3] Severity, duration, and recurrence of symptoms should be elicited, along with use of any products that contact the vulva and vagina. A sexual history should include a history of and risk factors for sexually transmitted infections (**Table 2**).

The pelvic examination starts with a careful external inspection. On speculum examination, characteristics of the vaginal mucosa (rugated or atrophic) and discharge are noted. Cervical friability, tenderness of the cervix, pain with palpation of the uterus, or presence of adnexal masses may indicate cervicitis or upper genital tract disease.[2]

Table 2
Patient history for vaginal complaints

Characteristic	Description
Discharge	Quantity Color Viscosity Relationship to menstrual cycle
Odor	Fishy or musty (bacterial vaginosis) Oniony (perspiration) Timing related to hour of day Timing related to bathing habits Clothing/underwear
Sensation felt	Itching Burning Irritation Acute, chronic or acute exacerbations of chronic sensation Combinations
Location	Vulva, vestibule or vagina
Dyspareunia	Acute or chronic Insertion vs deep thrust
Treatments	Antifungals, antibiotics, corticosteroids, or estrogen Topical, oral, or both Length of therapy for each course Response (complete resolution, partial resolution, or no response)
Irritants	Soaps, feminine hygiene products, douching Sensitizing agents such as benzocaine
Sexual history	Testing for sexually transmitted infections History of abuse or rape

In patients with long-term or recurring symptoms, additional physical examination elements may lead to the appropriate diagnosis (**Table 3**). Careful examination of the mouth for erosive lichen planus, axillae for hidradenitis suppurativa, and skin examination for fungal infection or acanthosis nigricans can reduce the difficulty of diagnosis.[2]

Table 3
Physical examination elements and testing for evaluation of vaginal symptoms

Area to Be Examined	Potential Findings
General	
Mouth	Reticular pattern of lichen planus, erosions, or ulcerations
Axilla and intertriginous areas	Pustules, cutaneous fungal infections, acanthosis nigricans
Pelvis	
Vulva and skin folds	Erythema, erosions, fissures, ulcers, masses, atrophy, alterations in vulvar architecture
Vestibular glands	Touch with a cotton swab for tenderness or erythema
Vagina	Discharge, erythema, inflammation, erosions, or synechiae
Cervix	Mucopurulent discharge or friability
Uterus	Tenderness

Laboratory Testing

Samples should be taken at the time of examination with the specific tests determined by the clinical scenario. For all patients, a sample of the discharge should be collected from that picked up on the speculum or using a swab in the posterior vagina for saline and (KOH) preparations. A sample for pH should be taken from the mid vagina.[5] Samples for bacterial culture, fungal culture, and nucleic acid amplification tests for gonorrhea, chlamydia, and trichomonas should be considered.[2]

The saline and 10% KOH wet preps are the main tests used for diagnosis of vaginitis. There are multiple ways to prepare the slides, but the most common is to place some discharge on a glass slide and add a drop of saline. Likewise, the same process is repeated with a drop of 10% KOH, because yeast are more commonly seen on the KOH slide.[3] The fishy (amine) odor of BV can be noted by performing a "whiff" test of the 10% KOH preparation. Coverslips are applied and a general inspection of the slide is performed on low power (100×). A power of 400× is the standard magnification used to evaluate vaginal samples and should be used for diagnosis.[3] Although an important test for office evaluation, the saline and KOH preps have some limitations in terms of sensitivity, specificity, and likelihood of disease given a positive or negative test.[3]

Findings like trichomonads, clue cells, yeast pseudohyphae or buds, presence or absence of *lactobacilli*, and presence of leukocytes are evaluated on the saline wet preparation. White blood cells on saline microscopy are nonspecific and can indicate trichomoniasis, vaginal candidiasis, atrophic vaginitis, bacterial vaginitis, cervicitis, or upper genital tract infection. Along with history and physical examination, these office-based tests are adequate to diagnose most patients with vaginal complaints. However, additional, more complex testing may be needed in some cases.

PHYSIOLOGIC DISCHARGE

Discharge found within a normal vagina comes from several origins. Mucus is produced by the periurethral, Skene's, and Bartholin glands, and the cervix. Because there are no mucosal cells in the vagina, the discharge is a transudate secreted through the vaginal epithelium and from the cervix. Physiologic discharge (also known as leukorrhea) is therefore a culmination of fluid, cells, and cellular debris. A normal woman of reproductive age not on hormone therapy will produce approximately 1 to 3 g of vaginal discharge per day.[9] Hormonal modification of vaginal discharge can be misinterpreted as infection, with clear discharge at ovulation and thicker, white discharge during other phases of the cycle. This misperception is common, and in a tertiary care program, 9% of referred patients with chronic vulvovaginal complaints were diagnosed with physiologic discharge.[14] Characteristics of physiologic vaginal discharge and common vaginitides are listed in **Table 4**. Results of office-based testing are listed in **Table 5**. Urinary incontinence can be excluded by giving phenazopyridine for 1 to 2 days and looking for a change in color of the vaginal discharge.[2]

The value of in-office measurement of pH cannot be emphasized enough, but it is frequently underused. The American College of Obstetricians and Gynecologists and the Centers for Disease Control and Prevention stress its importance and have incorporated it in their guidelines for evaluation.[5,7] The results of pH testing can drive the entire diagnostic process by reducing the number of potential diagnoses.[2] Limitations of pH testing can occur when there is contamination of the specimen. Gel used to lubricate the speculum may alter measurement of pH. Likewise, douching, semen, and intravaginal medications can also alter pH measurement.[3,5]

Table 4
Characteristics of physiologic discharge in reproductive age women

Characteristic	Description
Discharge	
Quantity	Variable, depending on phase of menstrual cycle
Color	Clear, white, or light gray
Consistency	Thin liquid to pasty
pH	Usually 3.8–4.2
Odor	None
Vaginal epithelium	Pink and rugated
Microscopy (saline preparation)	
Squamous cells	Homogeneous cytoplasm, nucleus is small, well-demarcated and centrally located, distinctive cell membrane
White blood cells	Fewer than 5/hpf (400× magnification)
Dominant bacteria	Rods of bacteria are individually free floating in the microscopic field

Adapted from Faro S. Healthy vaginal ecosystem. In: Vaginitis: differential diagnosis and management. New York: The Parthenon Publishing Group; 2004. p. 13–20.

Table 5
Testing for causes of vaginitis

Condition	Vaginal pH	Microscopy[a]	Amines	Current Gold Standard
Normal	<4.7	Normal squamous cells, few white blood cells, background bacillary flora	Negative	Clinical diagnosis
Vulvovaginal candidiasis	<4.7	Hyphae, blastospores	Negative	Yeast culture with speciation
Bacterial vaginosis	≥4.7	Clue cells, coccobacillary flora	Positive	Gram stain (Nugent score)
Trichomoniasis	Varies	Trichomonads	Variable	Trichomonas vaginalis NAAT
Atrophic vaginitis	≥4.7	Parabasal cells, decreased mixed flora	Negative	Maturation index
Desquamative inflammatory vaginitis	≥4.7	Parabasal cells, white blood cells	Negative	Clinical diagnosis
Cytolytic vaginosis	≤4.2	Abundant background bacillary flora, fragmented squamous cells	Negative	Clinical diagnosis

Abbreviation: NAAT, nucleic acid amplification test.
[a] Saline and 10% potassium hydroxide.
Adapted from Nyirjesy P. Management of persistent vaginitis. Obstet Gynecol 2014;124(6):1135–46; and Faro S. Cytolytic vaginosis. In: Vaginitis: differential diagnosis and management. New York: The Parthenon Publishing Group; 2004. p. 103–5.

VULVOVAGINAL CANDIDIASIS

About 75% of all women will develop a symptomatic vulvovaginal candidiasis at least once in their lives. One-half of all women will have sporadic recurrences, with about 8% having at least 4 episodes every year (chronic recurrent vulvovaginal candidiasis).[15] Over-the-counter antifungal medications are in the top 10 of all over-the-counter medications sold in the United States,[16] and more than $1.8 billion were spent in 1995 on medical treatment, time off, and travel expenses because of candida vaginitis, with an extrapolated estimate of $3.1 billion in 2014.[15]

Requirements for a symptomatic infection include colonization with a *Candida* species. This colonization occurs by local transport from the perineum and perianal areas, by digital introduction or sexual transmission.[2] The microorganism adheres to the vaginal epithelium. If germination occurs, it promotes vaginitis.[17] Colonization is present in normal women and occurs in 30% at any single time and in 70% over the course of 1 year. It is a transient asymptomatic event, most commonly from *Candida albicans*,[18] and cultures may be positive in asymptomatic individuals.

Factors associated with the transition from asymptomatic colonization to symptomatic infection are intrinsic to the host, the environment, host behavior, or related to the organism itself. Intrinsic host factors include diabetes, particularly with an increase in *Candida glabrata* infection.[19] It is suggested that glycosuria may contribute to colonization and infection.[20] Antibiotic use has long been associated with symptomatic infection and usually occurs in women who are already colonized.[21] Estrogen use increases colonization and infection with *Candida* species.[22] Patients who are immunosuppressed, particularly owing to steroid use, tend to have more symptomatic infections.[2] Behavioral factors such as orogenital sex can increase infections.[23] Contraceptive method may increase episodes of candidiasis. The use of oral contraceptive pills, an intrauterine device, or a diaphragm with spermicide for contraception has been associated with an increase in episodes.[24] About 20% of male partners are colonized on the penis, but treatment of the male partner to prevent vulvovaginal candidiasis is not recommended.[7]

Causative Organisms

C albicans is the strain that colonizes 98% of women and is the most common cause of uncomplicated and complicated cases.[18,24] It causes almost all acute uncomplicated cases and about 70% of complicated cases of recurrent vulvovaginal candidiasis. The remaining 30% are caused by *C glabrata*, *C parapsilosis*, or a rarer species.[25]

Signs and Symptoms

Symptoms of acute infection are a thick white discharge, itching, irritation, soreness, burning, external dysuria, and dyspareunia. Vulvar redness, swelling, fissures, or excoriations and vaginal erythema can be seen on physical examination, along with a thick discharge on speculum examination.[26]

Diagnostic Testing

Visualization of pseudohyphae and/or blastospores (buds) on saline or 10% KOH microscopy, or a positive fungal culture in a symptomatic woman is necessary for diagnosis.[5] Findings on office-based testing for vulvovaginal candidiasis are shown in **Table 5**. Unfortunately, the sensitivity of saline and KOH microscopy for yeast is about 40% to 80%.[27,28] Specific sensitivities and specificities of office testing are shown in **Table 6**. If clinical suspicion is for vulvovaginal candidiasis and microscopy is

Table 6
Accuracy of office tests for diagnosis of vaginal candidiasis

Test	Sensitivity (%)	Specificity (%)	Likelihood Ratio (95% Confidence Interval) Positive	Negative
Yeast seen with KOH	38–83	77–94	2.7 (1.4–4.9) to 6.5 (2.5–17)	0.51 (0.30–0.86) to 0.66 (0.47–0.92)
Yeast seen with saline	65	75	2.6 (1.5–4.6)	0.46 (0.26–0.83)
pH <4.5	59–96	23	0.77 (0.66–0.90)	1.8 (1.3–2.4)
pH <4.9	71	90	7.2 (3.4–15)	0.32 (0.17–0.61)
pH >5.0	77	35	Not reported	Not reported

Adapted from Anderson MR, Klink K, Cohrssen A. Evaluation of vaginal complaints. JAMA 2004:291(11);1368–79.

negative, then culture with speciation should be obtained. Newer, more costly tests are available for diagnosis such as a DNA homology probe[27,28] or a polymerase chain reaction (PCR) test.[29–31] The PCR test shows presence of the *Candida* genus, but species-specific tests are available. Although PCR methods are more sensitive than culture, they have not been shown to improve clinical care.[29]

Studies have shown that diagnosis by history and physical examination alone are not adequate to diagnose vulvovaginal candidiasis.[3] Additionally, avoiding patient self-diagnosis and phone diagnosis in women with chronic symptoms is recommended because the rate of misdiagnosis is significant.[5]

Uncomplicated Versus Complicated Candida Infections

Uncomplicated infections are most common and are defined as sporadic or infrequent episodes with mild to moderate symptoms in nonpregnant, healthy women.[5] These patients respond very well to antifungal therapy, with complete resolution of symptoms in 80% to 90%.[2] Five percent to 8% of patients have a prolonged course with a treatment failure, chronic symptomatic infection,[18] or rapid relapse after successful treatment.[26] Complicated infections are defined as 4 or more episodes per year, severe infection, non-*albicans* infections, or in patients with medical complications such as diabetes, immunocompromised state, debilitated status, or taking immunosuppressive agents.[5,7]

There are no clear risk factors for a complicated course in one-half of these women, but they do have an increased rate of vaginal *Candida* colonization.[32] The difference may be alteration of local immunoregulatory mechanisms or patients may have increased sensitivity to yeast with an enhanced inflammatory response to colonization resulting in symptomatic infection.[33] Strains of *Candida* have different levels of virulence, which can also affect the rate and severity of complicated infections. Species vary in the secretion of aspartate proteinases, proteases, phospholipases, and mycotoxins. These substances can inhibit phagocytic activity and suppress the local immune system in the vagina.[17] There may also be genetic factors that contribute to the development of a complicated course.[24]

Treatment

Therapy for vulvovaginal candidiasis can be given systemically or topically (**Table 7**).[5,7,34] In patients with uncomplicated infections, it is 80% to 90% effective.[7] Side effects are uncommon, but include burning and irritation for topical treatment and

Table 7
Therapy for vulvovaginal candidiasis

Uncomplicated vulvovaginal candidiasis	
Over-the-counter agents	
Clotrimazole 1% cream	5 g intravaginally for 7–14 d
Clotrimazole 2% cream	5 g intravaginally daily for 3 d
Miconazole 2% cream	5 g intravaginally daily for 7 d
Miconazole 4% cream	5 g intravaginally daily for 3 d
Miconazole 100 mg vaginal suppository	1 suppository intravaginally for 7 d
Miconazole 200 mg vaginal suppository	1 suppository intravaginally for 3 d
Miconazole 1200 mg vaginal suppository	1 suppository intravaginally for 1 dose
Tioconazole 6.5% ointment	5 g intravaginally for 1 dose
Prescription Agents	
Butoconazole 2% cream	5 g intravaginally for 1 dose
Terconazole 0.4% cream	5 g intravaginally for 7 d
Terconazole 0.8% cream	5 g intravaginally for 3 d
Terconazole 80 mg vaginal suppository	1 suppository intravaginally for 3 d
Fluconazole 100–200 mg tablet	1 dose
Complicated vulvovaginal candidiasis	
Severe infection	
Any topical azole	Intravaginally daily for 7–14 d
Fluconazole 100–200 mg tablet	2 doses, 72 h apart
Maintenance therapy	
Any topical azole	Intravaginally daily for 7–14 d
Fluconazole 100–200 mg tablet	2 doses, 72 h apart
THEN	
Fluconazole 100–200 mg tablet	Weekly for 6 mo
Candida glabrata infection	
Vaginal boric acid 600 mg in gelatin capsule	1 capsule intravaginally daily for 14 d
Candida parapsilosis infection	
Vaginal boric acid 600 mg in gelatin capsule	1 capsule intravaginally twice daily for 14 d
Fluconazole 200 mg tablet	Twice weekly for 4 wk

Data from Refs.[2,5,7]

gastrointestinal intolerance or headache for oral therapy.[5] In patients with complicated infections from *C albicans*, there is often resolution of symptoms after a course of antifungal therapy.[7] Unfortunately, 35% of complicated patients will have a recurrence within 1 month of treatment.[2] For patients with severe infection, either a 7 to 14 day course of topical azole or 2 doses of fluconazole 150 mg, 72 hours apart is recommended.[7] Adding the second dose of fluconazole increased the cure rate from 67% to 80% in a randomized, placebo-controlled trial looking at women with severe infection.[35]

In women with recurrent infection from *C albicans*, a favorable response is usually seen from topical azole or oral fluconazole therapy. However, episodic therapy does not achieve satisfactory symptom control. Achieving mycologic control with topical azole for 7 to 14 days or fluconazole 100 to 200 mg for 3 doses, every 3 days, is helpful. Then, suppressive therapy can be instituted. Oral fluconazole (100–200 mg) once weekly for 6 months is the regimen of choice. More than 90% of patients have no episodes of vulvovaginal candidiasis during suppressive therapy.[5] However, once maintenance therapy is completed, 30% to 50% of women will have recurrence.[7] Many clinicians will restart maintenance therapy if the pathogen remains *C albicans*. For women who are unable or unwilling to use fluconazole, miconazole 2% cream or clotrimazole 1% cream can be used twice weekly.[2] Patients who have had a positive culture for *C albicans* who do not respond to this regimen should have a repeat culture. Although resistance to azole therapy has been reported,[36] it is rare and sensitivities are not recommended.

C glabrata infections do not respond as well to azole therapy. Initial therapy is vaginal boric acid in a gelatin capsule, 600 mg daily for 14 days. About 70% of patients will be cured. The boric acid may cause local irritation or discharge, but is generally well-tolerated.[37] Flucytosine is the second line treatment, compounded into a 15.5% vaginal cream, 5 g daily for 14 days, but access to this medication is limited by cost.[37] Amphotericin B suppositories have been reported and could be another option for patients.[38]

A case series published by Nyirjesy and colleagues[39] described 17 of 19 patients with *C parapsilosis* who had negative cultures after fluconazole 200 mg twice weekly for 4 weeks and 6 of 6 patients who received boric acid vaginal capsules 600 mg twice daily for 2 weeks. Although these are limited data, they do present options for women with this rare infection.

Pregnant patients may be more susceptible to *Candida* species colonization and infection.[40] Higher dose fluconazole has been linked to birth defects; therefore, topical azole therapy for 7 days is indicated.[41]

BACTERIAL VAGINOSIS

BV is a polymicrobial infection and its hallmark feature is a lack of hydrogen peroxide-producing lactobacilli. Subsequently, there is an overgrowth of facultative anaerobic organisms.[5] Specific bacteria often found in patients with BV include *Gardnerella vaginalis, Mycoplasma homonis, Bacteroides* species, *Peptostreptococcus* species, *Fusobacterium* species, and *Prevotella* species, among others.[42] These bacterial species can be found among the normal flora of the vagina (see **Table 1**); therefore, it is the disruption of the vaginal ecosystem, not their mere presence that causes disease.

BV has been associated with additional morbidities in women. Low birth weight, premature rupture of membranes, and prematurity in pregnant women is increased in those BV.[43–45] Treatment is safe in pregnancy and effective at eradicating symptoms.[5] However, studies have shown conflicting conclusions as to whether routine screening and treatment of BV decreases the risk of preterm premature rupture of the membranes and preterm delivery.[5]

A number of infections such as pelvic inflammatory disease, postoperative gynecologic infections, and acquisition of human immunodeficiency virus (HIV) or herpes simplex virus (HSV) 2 infections are associated with BV in nonpregnant women. It is not known whether treatment of asymptomatic BV will decrease the risk of these infections; however, the treatment of BV before abortion or hysterectomy does decrease the risk of postoperative infection.[46,47]

Depending on the population studied, prevalence is between 9% and 37%.[48] About one-half are asymptomatic.[49] The population in this study showed that black and Hispanic women had a higher prevalence than white women (35% and 30% vs 27%;

$P = .02$).[48] Patients were more likely to have a history of gonococcal infection ($P = .04$) and trichomoniasis ($P = .02$), but a history of any sexually transmitted disease was not significant.[48] Sexual practices that increase the risk of BV include an increased frequency of intercourse, receptive oral sex, and a greater number of sexual partners.[49] Hormonal concentrations and shifts such as in pregnancy, with use of exogenous hormones, and the normal menstrual cycle also affect the normal flora and risk of BV.[49] Presence of a foreign body and use of medications such as antibiotics, douching agents, and spermicides also alter the vaginal ecosystem.[49] BV is not seen in premenarchal girls.

Signs and Symptoms

Symptoms of BV include abnormal vaginal discharge with a fishy odor.[5] Pruritus, irritation, and burning of the vulva are not seen in the typical BV case. The hallmark physical examination finding is a white/gray vaginal discharge that is seen on the vaginal sidewalls with speculum examination.

Diagnostic Testing

Amsel's criteria are used for office diagnosis of BV on saline wet preparation, and of the following 4 findings, 3 are required[50]:

1. Thin, homogeneous gray vaginal discharge,
2. Vaginal pH greater than 4.5,
3. Positive amine test ("whiff test"), and
4. Clue cells comprising greater than 20% of all squamous cells on saline microscopy.

The Nugent score is used for research on BV, and is considered the gold standard test. It is performed on a Gram stain and assigns a value to different bacterial types resulting in a score; a score of 7 or greater is considered positive for BV.[51] Other tests include point-of-care colorimetric testing that measures vaginal pH and volatile vaginal fluid amines. The use of colorimetric testing is no better or worse than 2 of 4 Amsel's criteria, and its routine use is not supported.[48] Finally, DNA testing by real-time PCR is available, which reports the presence or absence of *Lactobacillus* spp., *Atopobium vaginae, Megasphaera* spp., and *G vaginalis*.[52] This testing is costly and only detects the presence or absence of a few select bacteria associated with BV, which can be normal inhabitants of the vagina.[48] Cultures are not indicated.[2]

Recurrent Bacterial Vaginosis

There is no clear definition of recurrent BV, but certainly some women are troubled by the problem. After treatment, a single recurrence or more may occur in up to 58% of women within 12 months.[53] This study also showed that risk factors for recurrence included a history of BV, having a regular sex partner, or having a female sex partner.[53] Hormonal contraception was protective, most likely from the stable hormonal levels achieved.[53]

Vaginal biofilms have recently become a point of study for patients with recurrent BV compared with those who do not. Patients with *G vaginalis* and *A vaginae* had a much higher rate of recurrence at 1 year than those in whom *G vaginalis* alone was present (83% vs 38%; *P*<.001). Produced by bacteria, biofilms can coat surfaces allowing the microbes to hide from the effects of antibiotics. A recent study showed that 90% of women with and 10% of women without BV have a complex polymicrobial biofilm.[54] Standard treatment regimens may decrease the bacterial load, but not eliminate the biofilm, resulting in recurrence.[54] Longer treatment courses may improve resolution.

Because of the associations with sexual behavior, an argument for sexual transmission can be made. However, this has not been proven and data are limited. Some men have been shown to have a polymicrobial *G vaginalis*-dominant biofilm, which continues to incite debate.[2,54] Thus, recurrent BV could be a result of reinfection through sexual activity, failure to reestablish normal lactobacillus-dominant flora, or persistence of a vaginal biofilm.[2]

Treatment

Treatment of BV can be oral or topical (**Table 8**). All of the azole therapies have equivalent efficacy. Therapy can be individualized based on cost, side effects, and mode of administration. If treatment fails, the patient can often be cured with an additional course of the same therapy.[5,7]

For patients with recurrent BV, treatment of sexual partners has not shown a benefit and is not recommended.[2] Likewise, recolonization attempts with lactobacillus supplements are not recommended owing to a lack of evidence showing benefit.[2] Other recommendations such as condom use and cleaning of shared sex toys between uses seem logical and are not harmful, but have no scientific basis.[2]

Maintenance therapy with antibiotics has been studied and shown to be beneficial. Metronidazole gel given as an initial 10-day course with subsequent doses twice weekly for 4 months decreased recurrence compared with patients receiving placebo (26% vs 59%; $P = .001$). Unfortunately, 51% of patients recurred within 3 months and 59% of patients got vulvovaginal candidiasis.[55] Reichman and colleagues[56] used a regimen of metronidazole or tinidazole (500 mg) twice daily for 7 days, followed by 21 days of boric acid 600 mg vaginal suppositories, followed by twice weekly metronidazole gel for 16 weeks. The rates of cumulative cure at 12, 16, and 28 weeks were 87%, 78%, and 65%, respectively. However, the failure rate at 36 weeks was 50%.[56] Because of the high failure rate for long-term cure, more work is needed in this area.

Table 8 Treatment for acute bacterial vaginosis		
Medication	**Dose**	**Notes**
Metronidazole 500 mg Tablet	500 mg Twice Daily for 7 d	No alcohol consumption for until after 24 h from the last dose
Metronidazole 0.75% gel	5 g daily for 5 d	No alcohol consumption for until after 24 h from the last dose
Clindamycin 2% cream	5 g at bedtime for 7 d	May weaken latex or rubber condoms and diaphragms therefore, do not use until 5 d after the last treatment
Tinidazole 2 g tablet	2 g daily for 2 d	No alcohol consumption until after 5 d from the last dose
Tinidazole 1 g tablet	1 g daily for 5 d	No alcohol consumption until after 5 d from the last dose
Clindamycin 300 mg tablet	300 mg twice daily for 7 d	
Clindamycin 100 mg ovule	1 ovule at bedtime for 3 d	May weaken latex or rubber condoms and diaphragms therefore, do not use until 72 h after the last treatment

Adapted from Workowski KA, Bolan GA. Centers for Disease Control and Prevention. Sexually transmitted diseases treatment guidelines, 2015. MMWR Recomm Rep 2015;64(No. RR–3):69–77.

TRICHOMONAS VAGINITIS

Trichomonas affects an estimated 3.7 million persons in the United States.[57] It is much more common in black women (13%) than non-Hispanic white women (1.8%), representing a significant health disparity.[58] It is also more common in sexually transmitted disease (STD) clinic patients and incarcerated women.[7] Regardless of symptomatology, it is easily transmitted between partners during penile–vaginal intercourse,[59] and is best prevented with correct condom use. Sequelae of trichomonas infection includes a 2- to 3-fold increase in risk for HIV acquisition, preterm birth, low birth weight, and other adverse pregnancy outcomes in pregnant women.[5,7]

Signs and Symptoms

Symptomatic women complain of an abnormal vaginal discharge that is yellow-green, dyspareunia, vulvovaginal soreness and itching, and pain with urination.[2,5] However, 70% to 85% of infected persons have minimal or no symptoms.[5] Physical examination findings include vulvovaginal erythema, discharge, and occasionally punctate hemorrhages of the vaginal mucosa and cervix.[2]

Routine screening for all women seeking STD testing should be determined by the local epidemiology of *Trichomonas vaginalis* infection, because data are lacking on whether routine screening of asymptomatic women who are at high risk results in fewer adverse health events and health disparities.[7] However, routine screening is recommended in women with HIV because of an increased risk for pelvic inflammatory disease.[7]

The most commonly used diagnostic test is the wet mount, which has poor sensitivity (51%–65%).[60,61] Nucleic acid amplification testing is highly sensitive and detects RNA by transcription-mediated amplification. NAATs can be used on vaginal, endocervical, or urine specimens for women. Vaginal swab and urine have up to 100% concordance.[60] Point-of-care and patient self-testing are also viable options, and studies have shown that young women aged 14 to 22 years could correctly perform and interpret the self-test more than 99% of the time.[62]

Recurrent and Persistent Trichomonas Infections

Not all patients with trichomonas are straightforward. The most common reasons women have persistent or recurrent vaginitis are missed diagnosis (about one-third), metronidazole-resistant infection (about one-third), and incident cases occurring in women being treated for other conditions.[63] Persistent infections owing to treatment failure can be related to noncompliance, reinfection and metronidazole resistance, which occurs in 1.7% to 10.1%.[64] With treatment resistant infection, the Centers for Disease Control and Prevention guidelines recommend obtaining cultures for resistance testing and can help with management (telephone 404-718-4141; web site: http://www.cdc.gov/std).[7]

Treatment

Signs, symptoms, and possibly transmission of *T vaginalis* are reduced with treatment.[7] In women with HIV, adverse outcomes are reduced.[7] The nitroimidazoles are the only class of antimicrobial drugs known to be effective. Metronidazole and tinidazole are approved by the US Food and Drug Administration for this indication. Recommended regimens include:

- Metronidazole 2 g orally in a single dose,
- Tinidazole 2 g orally in a single dose, and
- Metronidazole 500 mg orally twice a day for 7 days (for women with HIV).

Metronidazole and tinidazole are equally efficacious for parasitologic cure (84% to 98% vs 92% to 100%).[5] Tinidazole has fewer gastrointestinal side effects than metronidazole, but is much more expensive, making metronidazole the therapy of choice for most women.[7] Metronidazole gel is much less efficacious than oral metronidazole and is not recommended for the treatment of *T vaginalis* infections.[7] In the case of immunoglobulin E-mediated–type allergy to nitroimidazoles, desensitization in consultation with an allergist is necessary.[2]

Patients should be advised to abstain from intercourse until they and their sex partners are treated and symptoms have resolved. All women with trichomonas should be tested for HIV and other STDs. Patients have a high rate of reinfection (17% in 3 months), so retesting for *T vaginalis* is recommended more than 2 weeks from treatment, even if they believe their sex partners were treated.[7] Concurrent treatment of all sex partners is essential to achieve symptomatic relief and microbiologic cure. Partners should be treated presumptively, and testing for trichomonas is not necessary. Expedited partner therapy is legal in some states, but is not superior to referral for treatment.[7] Side effects include a possible disulfiram-like effect, so alcohol should be avoided for 24 hours after metronidazole use and 72 hours after tinidazole.[5] Metronidazole is considered safe to use in pregnancy, but data on tinidazole are limited.[5]

For persistent or recurrent trichomonas infection, initial therapy is a longer course of metronidazole such as 500 mg orally twice daily for 7 days and, if necessary, metronidazole 2 g or tinidazole 2 g orally daily for 5 days. Another high dose regimen is tinidazole 1 g orally 2 to 3 times daily with 500 mg vaginally once daily for 14 days, resulting in cure for 92% of patients.[65] Additionally, paromomycin may have a place in treatment of trichomonal infections but data are limited.[2]

DESQUAMATIVE INFLAMMATORY VAGINITIS

DIV is an infrequent and severe form of purulent vaginitis, first described in 1965.[66] It occurs most commonly in perimenopausal white women.[67] The cause is unknown but disproved theories include estrogen deficiency, bacterial infection, or vitamin D deficiency.[66] In 1 study looking for a common bacterial pathogen, there was none found but there were some limitations to this study, namely, the inability to culture obligate anaerobic bacteria.[68] Current theories are that DIV is a noninfectious disease with a genetic predisposition for an abnormal immune attack on elements in the vaginal mucosa.[67]

Symptoms of DIV include a purulent vaginal discharge, severe dyspareunia, pruritus, or irritation.[67] On physical examination, there is a deep, fiery red erythema of the vagina and erosions with well-defined borders. The lesions appear in a spotted or linear pattern and ecchymosis can sometimes be seen.[66,67] The pH is greater than 5 and saline microscopy shows an increase in parabasal and inflammatory cells (neutrophils).[66] The inflammatory cell to squamous cell ratio is typically 1:1.[67] Dominance of Lactobacilli is not seen. See **Box 1** for a summary of the clinical characteristics of DIV. Yeast, trichomonas, other sexually transmitted diseases, and lichen planus must always be excluded before a diagnosis of DIV can be made.

Treatment is based on one of 2 approaches studied in the literature: topical corticosteroids or topical clindamycin. Steroid treatment with intravaginal corticosteroids, hydrocortisone 12.5 mg vaginal suppositories 2 times a day for 2 months, then daily for 2 months, then maintenance therapy 1 to 3 times per week has been shown to be effective.[69] Higher doses of hydrocortisone in a 10% cream are thought to be superior.[67] Women treated with 2% clindamycin intravaginal suppositories show initial improvement rates of 94%.[67] Interestingly, it may be owing to the antiinflammatory

---

Box 1
Clinical characteristics of desquamative inflammatory vaginitis

Postcoital bleeding

Dyspareunia

Pruritus

Purulent vaginal discharge

Irritation or burning, including the vestibule

Erosions in a spotted or linear pattern

Areas of hemorrhage or ecchymosis

Areas of a white reticulated pattern

pH ≥ 5

Lack of *Lactobacillus* predominance

Large numbers of squamous cells and parabasal cells

Large number of white blood cells (mostly neutrophils)

Adapted from Faro S. Desquamative vaginitis. In: Vaginitis: differential diagnosis and management. New York: The Parthenon Publishing Group; 2004. p. 99–102; and Sobel JD, Reichman O, Misra D, et al. Prognosis and treatment of desquamative inflammatory vaginitis. Obstet Gynecol 2011;117(4):850–5.

---

properties of macrolides with inhibition of cytokine synthesis.[67] Regardless of therapeutic regimen, cure rates (no evidence of disease off medication) are low (26% at 1 year) and another 58% were controlled (no evidence of disease on medication) at 1 year, but required maintenance therapy.[67] Patients in this study with a poor prognosis were more likely to have subsequent development of positive vaginal yeast cultures or to require therapy to the vestibule.[67] A chronic disease, DIV typically requires long-term therapy and careful attention to recurrent symptoms.

CYTOLYTIC VAGINOSIS

Cytolytic vaginosis occurs owing to an alteration in the vaginal ecosystem and is characterized by abundant overgrowth of *Lactobacilli*.[70,71] Normally, *Lactobacilli* block the adhesion of yeast organisms to the vaginal epithelium, but if overgrowth of *Lactobacilli* occurs, then the vaginal epithelium can be damaged, causing dissolution of the cells.[71] It is thought that the amount of *Lactobacilli* in the vagina varies according to the menstrual cycle, with the most being present in the luteal phase. Thus, cytolytic vaginosis can be at its symptomatic peak before menses and can recur with the menstrual cycle.[72]

Symptoms include pruritus, dyspareunia, and vulvar dysuria. The vulva seems to be normal without erythema. Vaginal discharge is white with a pasty appearance and the vaginal walls can be slightly erythematous. On office-based testing, the pH will be slightly lower than normal (3.5–4.5) and the wet preparation will show no clue cells, yeast, trichomonads, or leukocytes. Abundant lactobacilli are seen with fragmented squamous cells (see **Table 5**).[70]

Treatment is aimed at increasing the vaginal pH slightly to reduce the amount of *Lactobacilli*. Suggested treatment options are:

1. Sodium bicarbonate douching with 1 to 2 tablespoons of baking soda in 4 cups of warm water, used twice weekly for 2 weeks[71] and
2. Sodium bicarbonate–filled gelatin capsule placed intravaginally, twice weekly for 2 weeks.[71]

Treatment can be repeated as needed for an increase in symptoms.[72] Studies have shown that, in patients presenting for recurrent vulvovaginal candidiasis symptoms, cytolytic vaginosis is diagnosed in 5% to 7% of patients.[73,74] A high index of suspicion is needed to diagnose this condition and provide relief to these patients.

SUMMARY

Vaginal complaints are common and cause decreased quality of life in women. Relying on patient history, patient self-diagnosis, physical examination, or limited testing is ill-advised because these diagnostic methods have a high rate of misdiagnosis. Although most cases are uncomplicated and respond to a first-line therapeutic modality, some cases do not. A methodical, thorough approach will decrease the total time from onset of symptoms to diagnosis, and improve patient outcomes.

REFERENCES

1. Lipsky MS, Waters T, Sharp LK. Impact of vaginal antifungal products on utilization of health care service: evidence from physician visits. J Am Board Fam Pract 2000;13:178–82.
2. Nyirjesy P. Management of persistent vaginitis. Obstet Gynecol 2014;124(6): 1135–46.
3. Anderson MR, Klink K, Cohrssen A. Evaluation of vaginal complaints. JAMA 2004;291(11):1368–79.
4. Mulley AG. Approach to the patient with a vaginal discharge. In: Goroll AH, Mulley AG, editors. Primary Care medicine: office evaluation and management of the adult patient. Philadelphia: Lippincott Williams & Wilkins; 2000. p. 702–7.
5. Vaginitis. ACOG Practice Bulletin No. 72. American College of Obstetricians and Gynecologists. Obstet Gynecol 2006;107:1195–206.
6. American College of Obstetricians and Gynecologists. ACOG practice bulletin no. 93: diagnosis and management of vulvar skin disorders. Obstet Gynecol 2008;111:1243–53.
7. Workowski KA, Bolan GA, Centers for Disease Control and Prevention. Sexually transmitted diseases treatment guidelines, 2015. MMWR Recomm Rep 2015; 64(No. RR-3):69–77.
8. Sumawong V, Gregoire AT, Johnson WD, et al. Identification of carbohydrates in the vaginal fluid of normal females. Fertil Steril 1962;13:270–80.
9. Faro S. Healthy vaginal ecosystem. In: Vaginitis: differential diagnosis and management. New York: The Parthenon Publishing Group; 2004. p. 13–20.
10. Dahiya RS, Speck ML. Hydrogen peroxide formation by lactobacilli and its effect on Staphylococcus aureus. J Dairy Sci 1968;51:1068–72.
11. Mijac VD, Dukić SV, Opavski NZ, et al. Hydrogen peroxide producing lactobacilli in women with vaginal infections. Eur J Obstet Gynecol 2006;129:69–76.
12. Vásquez A, Jakobsson T, Ahrné S, et al. Vaginal lactobacillus flora of healthy Swedish women. J Clin Microbiol 2002;40(8):2746–9.
13. Aroutcheva A, Gariti D, Simon M, et al. Defense factors of vaginal lactobacilli. Am J Obstet Gynecol 2001;185(2):375–9.

14. Nyirjesy P, Peyton C, Weitz MV, et al. Causes of chronic vaginitis: analysis of a prospective database of affected women. Obstet Gynecol 2006;108(5):1185–91.
15. Foxman B, Barlow R, D'Arcy H, et al. Candida vaginitis: self-reported incidence and associated costs. Sex Transm Dis 2000;27:230–5.
16. Marrazzo JM. Vulvovaginal candidiasis. BMJ 2003;326:993–4.
17. Sobel JD. Vulvovaginal candidosis. Lancet 2007;369(9577):1961–71.
18. Beigi RH, Meyn LA, Moore DM, et al. Vaginal yeast colonization in nonpregnant women: a longitudinal study. Obstet Gynecol 2004;104:926–30.
19. de Leon EM, Jacober SJ, Sobel JD, et al. Prevalence and risk factors for vaginal Candida colonization in women with type I and type II diabetes. BMC Infect Dis 2002;2:1.
20. Nyirjesy P, Zhao Y, Ways K, et al. Evaluation of vulvovaginal symptoms and Candida colonization in women with type 2 diabetes mellitus treated with canagliflozin, a sodium glucose co-transporter 2 inhibitor. Curr Med Res Opin 2012;28:1173–8.
21. Pirotta MV, Garland SM. Genital Candida species detected in samples from women in Melbourne, Australia, before and after treatment with antibiotics. J Clin Microbiol 2006;44:3213–7.
22. Fischer G, Bradford J. Vulvovaginal candidiasis in postmenopausal women: the role of hormone replacement therapy. J Low Genit Tract Dis 2011;15:263–7.
23. Gieger AM, Foxman B. Risk factors for vulvovaginal candidiasis: a case-control study among university students. Epidemiology 1996;7:182–7.
24. Nyirjesy P. Vulvovaginal candidiasis and bacterial vaginosis. Infect Dis Clin North Am 2008;22:637–52, vi.
25. Nyirjesy P, Seeney SM, Grody MH, et al. Chronic fungal vaginitis: the value of cultures. Am J Obstet Gynecol 1995;173:820–3.
26. Eckert LO, Hawes SE, Stevens CE, et al. Vulvovaginal candidiasis: clinical manifestations, risk factors, management algorithm. Obstet Gynecol 1998;92:757–65.
27. Elie CM, Lott TJ, Reiss E, et al. Rapid identification of Candida species with species-specific DNA probes. J Clin Microbiol 1998;36:3260–5.
28. Lowe NK, Neal JL, Ryan-Wenger NA. Accuracy of the clinical diagnosis of vaginitis compared with a DNA probe laboratory standard. Obstet Gynecol 2009;113:89–95.
29. Sobel JD, Akins RA. The role of PCR in the diagnosis of Candida vulvovaginitis – a new gold standard? Curr Infect Dis Rep 2015;17:488.
30. Cartwright CP, Lembke BD, Ramachandran K, et al. Comparison of nucleic acid amplification assays with BD affirm VPIII for diagnosis of vaginitis in symptomatic women. J Clin Microbiol 2013;51:3694–9.
31. Weissenbacher T, Witkin SS, Ledger WJ, et al. Relationship between clinical diagnosis of recurrent vulvovaginal candidiasis and detection of Candida species by culture and polymerase chain reaction. Arch Gynecol Obstet 2009;279:125–9.
32. Giraldo P, von Nowaskonski A, Gomes FA, et al. Vaginal colonization by Candida in asymptomatic women with and without a history of recurrent vulvovaginal candidiasis. Obstet Gynecol 2000;95:413–6.
33. Fidel PL Jr, Barousse M, Espinosa T, et al. An intravaginal live Candida challenge in humans leads to new hypotheses for the immunopathogenesis of vulvovaginal candidiasis. Infect Immun 2004;72(5):2939–46.
34. Sobel JD, Brooker D, Stein GE, et al. Single oral dose fluconazole compared with conventional clotrimazole topical therapy of Candida vaginitis. Fluconazole Vaginitis Study Group. Am J Obstet Gynecol 2001;172:1263–8.

35. Sobel JD, Kapernick PS, Zervos M, et al. Treatment of complicated Candida vaginitis: comparison of single and sequential doses of fluconazole. Am J Obstet Gynecol 2001;185:363–9.
36. Marchaim D, Lemanek L, Bheemreddy S, et al. Fluconazole-resistant Candida albicans vulvovaginitis. Obstet Gynecol 2012;120:1407–14.
37. Sobel JD, Chaim W, Nagappan V, et al. Treatment of vaginitis caused by Candida glabrata: use of topical boric acid and flucytosine. Am J Obstet Gynecol 2003; 189:1297–300.
38. Phillips AJ. Treatment of non-albicans Candida vaginitis with amphotericin B vaginal suppositories. Am J Obstet Gynecol 2005;192:2009–12.
39. Nyirjesy P, Alexander AB, Weitz MV. Vaginal Candida parapsilosis: pathogen or bystander? Infect Dis Obstet Gynecol 2005;13:37–41.
40. Cotch MF, Hillier SL, Gibbs RS, et al. Epidemiology and outcomes associated with moderate to heavy Candida colonization during pregnancy. Vaginal Infections and Prematurity Study Group. Am J Obstet Gynecol 1998;178:374–80.
41. Xu J, Sobel JD. Candida vulvovaginitis in pregnancy. Curr Infect Dis Rep 2004;6: 445–9.
42. Ness RB, Hillier SL, Richter HE, et al. Douching is related to bacterial vaginosis, lactobacilli, and facultative bacteria in the vagina. Obstet Gynecol 2002;100: 765–72.
43. Gravett MG, Hummel D, Eschenbach DA, et al. Preterm labor associated with subclinical amniotic infection and with bacterial vaginosis. Obstet Gynecol 1986;67:229–37.
44. Hillier SL, Nugent RP, Eschenbach DA, et al. Association between bacterial vaginosis and preterm delivery of low-birth-weight infant. The Vaginal Infections and Prematurity Study Group. N Engl J Med 1995;333:1737–42.
45. Goldenburg RL, Hauth JC, Andrews WW. Intrauterine infection and preterm delivery. N Engl J Med 2000;342:1500–7.
46. Beigi RH, Austin MN, Meyn LA, et al. Antimicrobial resistance associated with the treatment of bacterial vaginosis. Am J Obstet Gynecol 2004;191:1124–9.
47. Koumans EH, Kendrick JS. Preventing adverse sequelae of bacterial vaginosis: a public health program and research agenda. CDC Bacterial Vaginosis Working Group. Sex Transm Dis 2001;28:292–7.
48. Gutman RE, Peipert JF, Weitzen S, et al. Clinical Diagnosis of bacterial vaginosis. Obstet Gynecol 2005;105(3):551–6.
49. Faro S. Bacterial vaginosis. In: Vaginitis: differential diagnosis and management. New York: The Parthenon Publishing Group; 2004. p. 25–35.
50. Amsel R, Totten PA, Spiegel CA, et al. Nonspecific vaginitis: diagnostic criteria and microbial and epidemiologic associations. Am J Med 1983;74:14–22.
51. Nugent RP, Krohn MA, Hillier SL. Reliability of diagnosing bacterial vaginosis is improved by a standardized method of Gram stain interpretation. J Clin Microbiol 1991;29:297–301.
52. Quest Diagnostics. SureSwab Bacterial Vaginosis DNA, Quantitative Real-Time PCR. Available at: http://www.questdiagnostics.com/testcenter/TestDetail.action? ntc=16898. Accessed August 16, 2016.
53. Bradshaw CS, Morton AN, Hocking J, et al. High recurrence rates of bacterial vaginosis over the course of 12 months after oral metronidazole therapy and factors associated with recurrence. J Infect Dis 2006;194:828–36.
54. Verstraelen H, Swidsinski A. The biofilm in bacterial vaginosis: implications for epidemiology, diagnosis and treatment. Curr Opin Infect Dis 2013;26:86–9.

55. Sobel JD, Ferris D, Schwebke J, et al. Suppressive antibacterial therapy with 0.75% metronidazole vaginal gel to prevent recurrent bacterial vaginosis. Am J Obstet Gynecol 2006;194:1283–9.
56. Reichman O, Akins R, Sobel JD. Boric acid addition to suppressive antimicrobial therapy for recurrent bacterial vaginosis. Sex Transm Dis 2009;36:732–4.
57. Satterwhite CL, Torrone E, Meites E, et al. Sexually transmitted infections among US women and men: prevalence and incidence estimates, 2008. Sex Transm Dis 2013;40:187–93.
58. Sutton M, Sternberg M, Koumans EH, et al. The prevalence of Trichomonas vaginalis infection among reproductive-age women in the United States, 2001-2004. Clin Infect Dis 2007;45:1319–26.
59. Sena AC, Miller WC, Hobbs MM, et al. Trichomonas vaginalis infection in male sexual partners: implications for diagnosis, treatment, and prevention. Clin Infect Dis 2007;44:13–22.
60. Hollman D, Coupey SM, Fox AS, et al. Screening for Trichomonas vaginalis in high-risk adolescent females with a new transcription mediated nucleic acid amplification test (NAAT): associations with ethnicity, symptoms, and prior and current STIs. J Pediatr Adolesc Gynecol 2010;23:312–6.
61. Roth AM, Williams JA, Ly R, et al. Changing sexually transmitted infection screening protocol will result in improved case finding for Trichomonas vaginalis among high-risk female populations. Sex Transm Dis 2011;38:398–400.
62. Huppert JS, Hesse E, Kim G, et al. Adolescent women can perform a point-of-care test for trichomoniasis as accurately as clinicians. Sex Transm Infect 2010;86:514–9.
63. Dan M, Sobel JD. Trichomoniasis as seen in a chronic vaginitis clinic. Infect Dis Obstet Gynecol 1996;4:77–84.
64. Krashin JW, Koumans EH, Bradshaw-Sydnor AC, et al. Trichomonas vaginalis prevalence, incidence, risk factors and antibiotic-resistance in an adolescent population. Sex Transm Dis 2010;37:440–4.
65. Sobel JD, Nyirjesy P, Brown W. Tinidazole therapy for metronidazole-resistance vaginal trichomoniasis. Clin Infect Dis 2001;33:1341–6.
66. Faro S. Desquamative vaginitis. In: Vaginitis: differential diagnosis and management. New York: The Parthenon Publishing Group; 2004. p. 99–102.
67. Sobel JD, Reichman OR, Misra D, et al. Prognosis and treatment of desquamative inflammatory vaginitis. Obstet Gynecol 2011;117(4):850–5.
68. Gardner HL. Desquamative inflammatory vaginitis: a newly defined entity. Am J Obstet Gynecol 1968;102:1102–5.
69. Mann MS, Kaufman RH. Erosive lichen planus of the vulva. Clin Obstet Gynecol 1991;34:605–13.
70. Faro S. Cytolytic vaginosis. In: Vaginitis: differential diagnosis and management. New York: The Parthenon Publishing Group; 2004. p. 103–5.
71. Suresh A, Rajesh A, Bhat R, et al. Cytolytic vaginosis: a review. Indian J Sex Transm Dis 2009;30(1):48–50.
72. Cibley LJ, Cibley LJ. Cytolytic vaginosis. Am J Obstet Gynecol 1991;165(4 Pt 2):1245–9.
73. Cerikcioglu N, Beksac MS. Cytolytic vaginosis: misdiagnosed as candida vaginitis. Infect Dis Obstet Gynecol 2004;12:13–6.
74. Wathne B, Holst E, Hovelius B, et al. Vaginal discharge comparison of clinical, laboratory and microbiological findings. Acta Obstet Gynecol Scand 1994;73:802–8.

Abnormal Uterine Bleeding
Current Classification and Clinical Management

Janice L. Bacon, MD, FACOG

KEYWORDS

- Abnormal uterine bleeding • Heavy menstrual bleeding • Intermenstrual bleeding

KEY POINTS

- Abnormal uterine bleeding (AUB) is now classified and categorized according to International Federation of Gynecology and Obstetrics guidelines.
- This applies to nongravid women during their reproductive years and allows more clear designation of causes, thus aiding clinical care and future research.
- These new categories are reviewed and current concepts of care are discussed.

The diagnosis and management of abnormal uterine bleeding (AUB) is one of the most common reasons women seek gynecologic care. Women with this complaint may have 1 or more conditions contributing to their symptoms. Medical terminology used to describe abnormal bleeding has had many descriptions and labels with poor correlation between the terminology and medical diagnosis, making research and clinical management of this spectrum of disorders difficult.

The International Federation of Gynecology and Obstetrics (FIGO) in 2005 convened an international committee of clinicians and investigators from 6 continents and more than 17 countries to propose a new classification for AUB. The first publication of this group addressed the standardization of terminology and definitions based on the characteristics of normal menstruation (**Box 1**).[1,2] The group decided that the 4 major clinical components of menstruation and the menstrual cycle would each be described by 3 simple words. These decisions were based on published data from the World Health Organization. Literature review yielded 6375 records of healthy women of reproductive age with normal menses with documentation of menstrual details and assisted with defining the characteristics of menses.[3] Normal menstrual volume was based primarily on research measures of hemoglobin loss in a Swedish

Disclosure Statement: The author has nothing to disclose.
Women's Health and Diagnostic Center, 2728 Sunset Boulevard, Lexington Medical Park One Suite 106, West Columbia, SC 29169, USA
E-mail address: jlbacon@lexhealth.org

Box 1
Characteristics of normal menstruation

Duration of flow: 4.5 to 8.0 days

Frequency (interval): 24 to 38 days (22–35 days in midreproductive years)

Cycle-to-cycle variation: ± 2 to 20 days (over 12 months)

Volume of blood loss: 5 to 80 mL

Menstrual terminology

Duration: prolonged, normal, shortened

Frequency: frequent, normal, infrequent

Regularity: regular, irregular, absent

Volume: heavy, normal, light

Data from Fraser IS, Critchley HO, Munro MG, et al. A process designed to lead to international agreement on terminologies and definitions used to describe abnormalities of menstrual bleeding. Fertil Steril 2007;87(3):466–76; and Fraser IS, Critchley HO, Munro MG, et al. Can we achieve international agreement on terminologies and definitions used to describe abnormalities of menstrual bleeding? Hum Reprod 2007;22(3):635.

---

community.[4] The concept of "menstrual shape" was discussed by the study group and it is "the patient's perception of the pattern of changes in normal volume from day to day."[1] This topic has had little study but may in the future be incorporated into the menstrual history.

The FIGO group agreed to abandon the term dysfunctional uterine bleeding (DUB) and replace the term menorrhagia with "heavy menstrual bleeding (HMB)." AUB may describe abnormal HMB or mistimed bleeding, and it may be acute or chronic. The 2009 FIGO workgroup suggested defining acute AUB as "an episode of heavy bleeding that, in the opinion of the clinician, is of sufficient quantity to require immediate intervention to prevent further blood loss." Chronic AUB is defined as "bleeding from the uterine corpus that is abnormal in volume, regularity and/or timing and has been present for the majority of the past 6 months"; thus, it would not require immediate medical attention. Acute AUB could occur as a part of or within the occurrence of chronic AUB.[5] Intermenstrual bleeding (IMB) "occurs between clearly defined cyclic and predictable menses"[5] and replaces the term metrorrhagia. These occurrences may appear randomly or at a regular time in each cycle.

The FIGO classification system is divided into 9 categories. These divisions pertain to general clinical care. Subclassification could be used for research or subspecialty applications.[5] The 9 categories are arranged in the acronym PALM-COEIN ("palm-koin") (**Table 1**). The prior term "dysfunctional uterine bleeding (DUB)" was a diagnosis used when no systemic or anatomic cause for AUB was identified. This new system recognizes that any patient may have 1 or more entities contributing to abnormal bleeding or identified in the context of abnormal bleeding but remain asymptomatic. When AUB is caused by medical hormonal therapies, including intrauterine devices, it falls in the iatrogenic category. The "not yet classified" category encompasses rare or ill-defined disorders. Malignant/hyperplasia is a major category representing hyperplasia with and without atypia as well as malignancies of the uterine corpus. Malignancies are further categorized by World Health Organization (WHO) and FIGO classification and staging systems.

Table 1			
FIGO Classification system for AUB			
Discrete Structural Entities[a]			**Nonstructural Entities**
P	Polyp	C	Coagulopathy
A	Adenomyosis	O	Ovulatory dysfunction
L	Leiomyoma	E	Endometrial
M	Malignancy/Hyperplasia	I	Iatrogenic
		N	Not yet classified

Abbreviations: AUB, abnormal uterine bleeding; FIGO, Federation of Gynecology and Obstetrics.
  [a] Structural entities may be imaged or defined histopathologically.
From Munro MG, Critchley HO, Broder MS, et al. FIGO Classification System (PALM-COEIN) for causes of abnormal uterine bleeding in nongravid women of reproductive age. Int J Gynaecol Obstet 2011;113(1):5; with permission.

ENDOMETRIAL AND ENDOCERVICAL POLYPS

Cervical polyps (AUB-P) may arise from the cervix itself, may be a prolapsed endometrial polyp, or even a leiomyoma appearing in the cervical canal or at the external os. The etiology of true cervical polyps is unknown, although hormonal or inflammatory functions may play a role. Cervical polyps commonly occur in the later reproductive years (> age 40). They may have variable size and color. Histologically, cervical polyps are composed of vascular connective tissue surrounded by squamous, columnar, or squamo-columnar epithelium. Removal is recommended when large (>3 cm), symptomatic, or abnormal in appearance. Removal by grasping and twisting is usually simple. Cauterization or coagulation of the base may decrease recurrence. Malignancy is rare.[6]

Endometrial polyps are common causes of AUB in women before and after menopause. Histologically they are a hyperplastic growth of endometrial glands and stroma forming a projection from the surface of the endometrium and containing a vascular core and occasionally smooth muscle cells. The prevalence of endometrial polyps rises with increasing age. Their appearance may be pedunculated or sessile (broad based). Although many endometrial polyps are detected due to AUB, others are asymptomatic and found during imaging for other indications. Malignancy is occasionally noted.[7]

The cause of polyp formation is unknown, but they have been found to contain both estrogen and progesterone receptors.[8] Progesterone may have an antiproliferative effect on polyps, as it does on the endometrium, whereas endogenous or exogenous estrogen may be a risk factor. Cellular mechanisms proposed in the development of polyps include monoclonal abnormal hyperplasia,[9] overexpression of endometrial aromatase,[10,11] and gene mutations.[12,13]

Clinical risk factors for development of endometrial polyps include obesity, tamoxifen use, postmenopausal hormone therapy, and patients with Lynch or Cowden syndrome.

Although the most common clinical symptom of an endometrial polyp is AUB (reported as IMB in premenopausal women, postmenopausal bleeding, or breakthrough bleeding in menopausal women on hormone therapy). In women with endometrial cells on a cervical cytology report, 12% of the women had endometrial polyps, 72% of these were asymptomatic, whereas 2% of the polyps had other findings, such as endometrial hyperplasia.[14] Polyps are commonly identified by imaging or by hysteroscopy. Ultrasound may be enhanced by sonohysterography. Differentiation of polyps versus myomas may be based on ultrasound appearance, shadowing, and vascularity. Although a small number of polyps will regress, lesions larger than 1 cm are less likely to spontaneously resolve.[15]

Polyps are benign in 99% of cases.[16] A greater risk of malignancy is noted in postmenopausal women, polyps found during the evaluation of AUB, women on tamoxifen, or in women with polyps larger than 1.5 cm. Although polyps are not associated with pregnancy loss, removal may be best in women undergoing therapy for infertility.

There are no guidelines for management of a woman with an asymptomatic polyp who does not undergo polypectomy. The overall risk of recurrence of polyps is small. The Levonorgestrel Intrauterine System (LNG-IUS), Mirena, has been shown to decrease the recurrent risks of polyps particularly in women on tamoxifen.[17]

ADENOMYOSIS

Adenomyosis (AUB-A) is a condition in which endometrial glands and stroma reside in the uterine myometrium, inducing hypertrophy locally or throughout the uterine fundus and eventually causing enlargement of the uterine corpus. Localized areas may be difficult to distinguish from leiomyoma. The incidence of adenomyosis is reported to occur in 20% to 65% of women and is associated with increasing age. It has been reported in small numbers of adolescent women. Adenomyosis is commonly noted in association with leiomyoma, endometriosis, and early menarche.[18] Other articles have cited an association with severe dysmenorrhea, depression, and even prior uterine surgery.[19]

The etiology of adenomyosis is undetermined, but theories include invagination of the endometrium, de novo müllerian rests, or a metaplastic process. Altered molecular function of endometriotic glands or the junctional zone of the endometrium with the myometrium, as well as estrogen and progesterone, are also suggested etiologic factors. Pituitary hormones, prolactin and follicle-stimulating hormone, may be contributing influences. Some evidence suggests leiomyomas and adenomyosis may share a common origin in angionesis and growth factor dysregulation. Adenomyosis does not share pathogenic similarities with endometriosis other than the similar presenting symptom of pelvic pain.[20]

Physical and pathologic findings in uteri containing adenomyosis include gross enlargement and a "boggy" feel with the uterine volume and weight above normal parameters. Adenomyomas at imaging may appear similar to leiomyomas but do not exhibit discreet capsular formation and are not easily resected ("shelled out"). Histopathology features endometrial tissue 1 to 2 low-power fields from the endomyometrial junction.

Prominent clinical symptoms include HMB with dysmenorrhea or chronic pelvic pain, although up to 30% of women are asymptomatic. Confirmatory diagnosis requires a hysterectomy specimen, but ultrasound examination or MRI imaging revealing increased uterine volume, thickened myometrium, myometrial cysts, or increased myometrial heterogeneity with loss of a clear endometrial myometrial junction are highly suggestive of this disorder.

Although hysterectomy is the only definitive treatment for adenomyosis, hormonal therapy is effective for many women. Therapeutic options include combination oral contraceptives (estrogen and progesterone), progesterone-only therapy, gonadotropin-releasing hormone (GnRH) agonists, or aromatase inhibitors. The most promising progesterone therapy is the LNG-IUS.[20] Hormonal therapies not only reduce menstrual volume but dysmenorrhea as well.

Procedures aside from hysterectomy have included endometrial ablation or resection, excision of adenomyomas, or laparoscopic myometrial electrocoagulation.

Surgical intervention with postoperative medical therapy may be better than surgery alone.[21] A few reports of uterine artery embolization or MRI-guided focused ultrasound surgery have shown some promise.[22,23] Hysterectomy remains the therapy of choice for women who have completed child bearing.

LEIOMYOMATA

Leiomyomas (AUB-L) are common fibromuscular tumors of the myometrium with a high prevalence in women[24]; the large variation in size, location, and number requires subclassification within this FIGO category. Many are asymptomatic and others have varying rates of growth and secondary symptoms. The FIGO system proposes classification of fibroids by location. Fibroids may have 1 or more classifications due to the size of the fibroid and therefore its impact on more than 1 site in the uterus. The 3 large subgroups are intermural, submucosal, and subserosal. Leiomyomas also may involve the broad ligament or cervix.

Uterine leiomyomas are benign monoclonal tumors from the smooth muscle myometrium surrounded by a pseudocapsule of areolar tissue and compressed muscle fibers. The most likely etiology is normal myocytes transformed into abnormal myocytes that then grow into clinically apparent tumors. Many factors, such as steroid hormones, environment, genetics, and growth factors related to angiogenesis and fibrotic processes, contribute to growth and clinical manifestations.[25] Excessive uterine bleeding related to uterine fibroids is thought to be caused by changes in the endometrium and its vasculature.[26,27] Sixty percent of leiomyoma have abnormal karyotypes and some of these are seen more frequently: trisomy 12, translocation between chromosomes 12 and 14, and chromosome deletions or rearrangements.[28] Some women may have a family predisposition to leiomyoma.[29]

Steroid hormones have a complex relationship to leiomyoma. Estrogen and progesterone and their receptors are involved in fibroid pathogenesis as well as aromatase and even stem cells. Molecular changes leading to increased angiogenic growth factors and thus abnormal blood vessel number and function, are suggested to play a role in fibroid-associated symptoms as well as dysregulated fibrotic growth factors.[26]

Risk factors for the development of leiomyomas include race (black greater than white), early menarche, hypertension, obesity, and dietary factors. Higher parity or shorter pregnancy intervals and tobacco smoking may reduce risks. Hormonal contraceptives and ovulation-inducing agents appear neutral. Investigations of vitamin sufficiency or insufficiency and the role of uterine infections are ongoing.

The most commonly reported symptoms associated with leiomyoma are HMB, pelvic pressure or pain, and reproductive dysfunction. Bleeding may be heavy or prolonged but myomas are not associated with IMB or postmenopausal bleeding. Leiomyoma altering the endometrial cavity or protruding into the endometrial cavity are most associated with HMB and increase the risk of anemia. Large fibroid bulk may be associated with urinary frequency, difficulty emptying the bladder, or constipation. Dysmenorrhea has been reported and dyspareunia may be associated with anterior or fundal myomas. The presence of fibroids may increase the risk of miscarriage, decrease conception rate, or cause pregnancy complications, including fetal growth restriction, placental abruption, malpresentation, and preterm labor.

The physical and bimanual examination are the most important first-line evaluations of the uterus, assessing uterine size and contour. Imaging aids the evaluation of fibroids: number, size, and location. Imaging modalities include transvaginal or abdominal ultrasound, diagnostic hysteroscopy, MRI, and hysterosalpingogram. Postmenopausal bleeding or abnormal bleeding may prompt endometrial sampling to rule out hyperplasia or malignancy as a process separate from the presence of the fibroids.

Some fibroids may be managed expectantly, especially those that are found without the presence of symptoms, but no specific guidelines exist. An imaging study at the time of diagnosis clarifies the absence of adnexal masses and allows documentation of leiomyoma number, size, and location. Annual examinations with interim evaluation if symptoms develop allow some patients to be followed conservatively.

In women with HMB, anemia must be assessed and other causes of anemia excluded.

Combination steroid hormones or progestin-only hormonal therapy may assist symptom management of HMB, but do not provide long-term treatment of the leiomyoma. The LNG-IUS observational studies and systemic reviews indicate a potential decrease in uterine volume and bleeding while providing excellent contraception. No randomized clinical trials are available at this time.[30,31]

GnRH agonists are the most effective medical therapy for leiomyomata, producing both amenorrhea and relief of fibroid symptoms with a 35% to 60% reduction in uterine size. Rebound symptoms occur when GnRH agonists are discontinued. Long-term use of GnRH agonists may not be desirable due to effects on bone density as well as menopausal symptoms, myalgias or arthralgias. The most common use of GnRH agonists is preoperatively to assist with increasing the patient's hematocrit.

Other medical agents considered for fibroid management include GnRH antagonists and progestin receptor modulators (none available in the United States). Ulipristal acetate (a progestin receptor modulator) and mifepristone (an antiprogesterone) hold future promise, although dosages suitable for long-term use are not currently determined. Endometrial changes caused by antiprogestins may appear as cystic glandular dilation with both estrogen and progesterone effects. Hyperplasia, however, does not occur, although the endometrium may appear thickened on ultrasound. Other medications that have been considered for medical management of symptomatic fibroids include raloxifene and aromatase inhibitors.

Surgical therapy has been the traditional treatment for leiomyomas: indications include symptomatic or bulky myoma, HMB, infertility, or recurrent pregnancy loss. Hysterectomy is indicated for women who have completed childbearing and are at risk for associated conditions, including neoplasia of the cervix, uterus, or ovaries or those women with endometriosis, adenomyosis, or failed conservative therapy (medical or surgical) who desire definitive treatment. A sizable myoma that is submucosal or subserosal may still be managed with myomectomy, but future risk for development for other leiomyomas remains. Hysteroscopic, laparoscopic, and robotic approaches have allowed myomectomy to be performed less invasively.

Endometrial ablation has performed poorly in women with submucous or intramural myomas, whereas laparoscopic myolysis by thermal, radiofrequency, or cryoablation, is under investigation. Uterine artery embolization or uterine fibroid embolization has performed well for women who wish to preserve their uterus but who have completed childbearing. It results in significant fibroid shrinkage with less pain and a shorter hospital stay than hysterectomy.[32] Unfortunately, these procedures have resulted in more complications and readmissions than hysterectomy and success is reduced in the presence of multiple leiomyomas or greater overall uterine size.[33] Long-term success is less and other interventions may be required if embolization is performed.[34]

A newer technique targeting individual myomas is magnetic resonance–guided focused ultrasound (MRgFUS). This is a noninvasive ultrasound thermal ablation technique. Food and Drug Administration labeling for this device now allows treatment in some women who wish to consider future childbearing. Success may be limited by fibroid number, calcified myomas, and individual fibroid vascularity, or by other uterine features, such as adenomyosis. This technique often results in a reduced myoma volume of approximately 40%.[35] Determination of optimal conditions for MRgFUS and long-term outcomes are needed. There are no comparison studies of this method with other minimally invasive techniques.

Few guidelines for clinicians comprehensively discuss all fibroid treatments. Those from the Royal College of Obstetricians and Gynecologists and the Society of Obstetricians and Gynecologists Canada provide treatment guidelines, but the most comprehensive recommendations are from France or the European Menopause and Andropause society, which do address integration of both medical and surgical approaches.[36–39]

MALIGNANCY AND HYPERPLASIA

This section discusses malignancy and hyperplasia (AUB-M). The WHO classification of endometrial hyperplasia (EH) is based on 4 etiologies:

1. Simple without atypia.
2. Complex without atypia.
3. Simple with atypia.
4. Complex with atypia.

The endometrial intraepithelial neoplasia classification system was an alternative proposed by an international group of gynecologic pathologists in 2000. It does not correspond directly with WHO guidelines but shows better intraobserver reproducibility and may be better at predicting progression to malignancy.[40]

In premenopausal or postmenopausal women with abnormal bleeding, malignancy must be excluded. The glandular and stromal architectural pattern determines the diagnosis of hyperplasia. The highest incidence of endometrial hyperplasia without atypia is seen in women ages 50 to 54 versus the highest incidence of EH with atypia is seen more commonly in ages 60 to 64.[41]

Risk factors for EH are similar to those risk factors for endometrial carcinoma (EC) and generally involve unopposed estrogen exposure. Specific risk factors include increasing age, obesity, early menarche, late menopause (older than 55), polycystic ovary syndrome, diabetes mellitus, nulliparity, tamoxifen therapy, or family history of EC or Lynch or Cowden Syndrome. EH in women who have an estrogen-producing tumor or who are estrogen deficient is especially worrisome for a malignant process. Presenting symptoms of EH are most commonly AUB or postmenopausal bleeding and less frequently the finding of endometrial cells on cervical cytology.

Diagnosis is made by examination and endometrial sampling with or without imaging, such as transvaginal ultrasound. Insufficient cells at the time of endometrial sampling warrants repeat sampling by endometrial biopsy or dilation and curettage. The differential diagnosis includes endometrial polyps or leiomyomata. The diagnosis of atypia in EH is most concerning for malignancy. Neither endometrial biopsy nor endometrial curettage, however, may be completely sufficient to exclude malignancy.[42] Oncologic consultation is often considered for the management of these patients.

For women who desire future childbearing, progesterone therapy is the most important treatment for prevention of future malignancy and continued abnormal bleeding. Progesterone options include the following:

1. Norethindrone acetate 5 to 15 mg daily 12 to 14 days per month.
2. Medroxy-progesterone acetate oral 10 mg daily for 3 to 6 months or 10 mg daily 12 to 14 days per month.

3. Depo Medroxyprogesterone acetate 150 mg intramuscularly every 3 months.
4. Levonorgestrel Intrauterine System (LNG-IUS).
5. Micronized Progesterone 100 or 200 mg for 12 to 14 days per month (oral or vaginal).
6. Combined oral contraceptives.[40]

Some of these regimens provide excellent contraception, but for women actively seeking pregnancy, ovulation induction increases endogenous progesterone production in the corpus luteum as well as assisting conception.

Regression of EH has been documented with expectant management or treatment in 70% to 85% of women.[43] Endometrial biopsy (EMB) should be repeated every 3 to 6 months until regression of hyperplasia is documented. If EH recurs, progestin dosage may be adjusted or the LNG-IUS may be considered. If atypia develops, a reappraisal of treatment with consultation from a gynecologic oncologist is appropriate.

When disease regression is documented, preventive measures should be instituted or regular menses documented. Alteration of hormone therapy in postmenopausal women or expectant management may be considered. If abnormal bleeding develops, endometrial sampling is required. Other medications under consideration for therapy for women who desire future childbearing include Danazol, GnRH agonist or antagonist, aromatase inhibitors. Hysteroscopic resection is under research.

COAGULOPATHY

Coagulopathy (AUB-C) is a term that describes a systemic disorder of hemostasis that manifests as AUB or HMB or simply contributes to these entities when other conditions are present. Women who require lifelong anticoagulation are also placed in this category, although their management and subsequent irregular bleeding could be considered iatrogenic. The new FIGO classification states it is more appropriate to place anticoagulated women in the coagulopathy category.

One in 5 women with HMB have a bleeding disorder. The most common diagnosis is von Willebrand disease, which affects 1% of the population.[44] The mildest form is the most frequently diagnosed. The next most common group of coagulopathies are platelet function defects. Factor deficiencies and hemophilia are much less frequent.

Noninherited causes of coagulopathy include acquired platelet dysfunction (nonsteroidal anti-inflammatory drug use, renal disease), idiopathic thrombocytopenia purpura, or acquired factor consumption. Historical questions that may provide clues to the presence of a coagulopathy are listed in **Box 2**.

Box 2
Historical questions to assist identification of a coagulopathy

1. History of bleeding problems (posttrauma, postoperative, postpartum)

2. History of iron-responsive anemia

3. History of transfusion

4. Ingestion of diet supplements, or medications that predispose to vitamin K deficiency

5. Thyroid disorders, renal disease, or liver dysfunction

6. Mucosal bleeding: epistaxis or gingival

7. Petechiae or ecchymosis

8. Heavy menstrual bleeding or intermenstrual bleeding

HMB is often difficult to define clinically, but is commonly identified in research studies as loss of more than 80 mL of blood per menses. Clinical clues to this diagnosis include menstrual flow lasting more than 7 days, soaked sanitary supplies more frequently than every hour, clots larger than 1 inch, or frequent soiling of clothing. Testing for specific causes of coagulopathy are listed in **Box 3**.

Coagulation factors may be affected by other medical conditions, including thyroid disorders, renal disease or abnormal liver function, active bleeding, prescription medications or hormone therapy, over-the-counter medications, or dietary supplements. Anatomic causes of the abnormal bleeding must be excluded.

Acute bleeding with decreased hemoglobin should prompt testing for a coagulopathy. Management may require combined estrogen and progesterone contraceptive regimens or even intravenous conjugated estrogens with tapering of a combined contraceptive regimen after bleeding is controlled. Laboratory tests for coagulopathy are preferably drawn before transfusion, because unstable patients may require hormone therapy and blood products. Occasionally surgical intervention with dilatation and curettage and balloon tamponade are needed. Procedures such as uterine artery embolization with nonpermanent gel foam may also be a management option, but care should be taken to avoid procedures that would preclude future pregnancy in young women of childbearing age or adolescents. Procedures associated with permanent loss of childbearing include endometrial ablation, UAE with permanent microspheres, and hysterectomy. **Table 2** lists options for hormonal management of acute menstrual bleeding.

Box 3
Testing for specific causes of coagulopathy

Initial Testing for Coagulopathies:

1. Complete blood count

2. Prothrombin time, partial thromboplastin time

3. Fibrinogen

4. Von Willebrand panel (von Willebrand factor antigen level, Ristocetin cofactor, factor VIII level)

Additional specific tests:

1. Peripheral blood smear

2. Platelet aggregation study (adenosine diphosphate, epinephrine collagen)

3. Platelet aggregometry

4. Coagulation factor assays

5. Clot solubility testing

6. Tests of fibrinogen function (Fibrin Split Products, D-dimer level)

Individualized assays for rare bleeding disorders:

1. Alpha-2-antiplasmin activity

2. Euglobulin clot lysis time

3. Tissue plasminogen activator level

4. Plasminogen activator inhibitor-1 analysis

Table 2
Hormonal therapies for acute abnormal uterine bleeding

Intravenous conjugated estrogens	25 mg Premarin every 4–6 h × 24 h (then institute combined hormone therapy)
Combined oral contraceptives (monophasic 35-μg pill)*	1 tab 3 times a day for 7 d, then taper
Oral norethindrone acetate	5–10 mg every 4 h until bleeding stops, then taper
Oral medroxyprogesterone acetate	10–40 mg every 4 h until bleeding stops, then taper

* Estrogen-containing regimens may increase the risk for clotting if predisposing conditions are present.

In addition to hormonal intervention, antifibrinolytics may assist control of bleeding. Transfusion ideally replaces needed blood products, although packed red blood cells may be started in unstable patients. A transfusion protocol may assist management for acute emergent blood loss.

Ovulatory Function

Ovulatory dysfunction (AUB-O) may manifest in a variety of patterns ranging from amenorrhea to variable flow at irregular intervals to HMB, thus falling outside the parameters listed for "ovulatory" cycles. These events can occur occasionally throughout the reproductive years but are more frequent near menarche and in the perimenopausal years. The etiology varies from medical or endocrine disorders to occasional events of uncertain etiology. Other potential causes of bleeding in ovulatory patients include infection or trauma. Anatomic abnormalities should be excluded. Prescription hormonal regimens or medications affecting the hypothalamic-pituitary-ovarian (HPO) axis and associated with irregular bleeding are termed iatrogenic, but FIGO has placed these events in the category of ovulatory dysfunction. Laboratory studies should exclude pregnancy and focus on the differential diagnosis for the individual patient's clinical presentation.

Anovulation is the primary etiology for AUB in adolescent women. The immature HPO axis is associated with unpredictable noncyclic bleeding, especially in the first 12 to 18 months after menarche. Three to 5 years after menarche, most young women have menstrual intervals of 21 to 34 days.[1] Bleeding episodes that are excessive in flow or occurrence may often prompt medical intervention and occasionally result in emergent acute bleeding. Several disorders encompassing different FIGO categories are diagnosed commonly in young women near menarche, including endocrine disorders, coagulopathies, and polycystic ovary syndrome. The rising incidence of obesity has increased the AUB-O diagnosis.

In women ages 19 to 39, endocrine disorders, particularly androgen excess disorders with secondary obesity as a cofactor, are a common etiology of AUB. These patients also comprise a group at risk for EH and even malignancy (AUB-M). Hormonal control of menses that provides contraception or ovulation induction in women desiring conception represent the most common therapeutic options.

After age 40, AUB-O is most commonly associated with the transition to menopause and declining ovarian function. Perimenopause begins with cycle irregularity and lasts until 1 year after the last menstrual period. Once pregnancy is excluded, hormonal contraception for women with no contraindications provides protection against unplanned pregnancy and relieves perimenopausal symptoms. EH and malignancy must be excluded, as well as checking for endometrial polyps or leiomyomata. Medical therapy is the first line of treatment, with surgery for those who fail medical management, are unable to tolerate medication, or who have significant anatomic abnormalities. Medical management of AUB-O has a wide range of choices, most of which are also excellent contraceptives (**Table 3**).

Surgical intervention by endometrial ablation (EAB) or hysterectomy may be offered to women who are not appropriate candidates for medical therapy. Endometrial ablation, however, does not provide contraception and poses significant risk to pregnancy if contraception is not prescribed. In addition, ablation techniques may limit future evaluation for EH or malignancy and may require hysterectomy for recurrent abnormal bleeding. Long-term complications of EAB include uterine synechiae, cervical stenosis, endometrial distortion, and delayed detection of endometrial malignancy.[45,46] EAB treats AUB without addressing the root cause of abnormal bleeding. Patients with risk factors for malignancy may be at actual increased risk from delayed diagnosis.

Endometrial

In women with regular cyclic menses who have AUB but no other identified cause, a disorder of the endometrium is possible (AUB-E). HMB in this setting may be a disorder of local endometrial "hemostasis." This would evolve due to decreased local production of vasoconstrictor, prostaglandin F2 alpha, and endothelin-1, and/or accelerated lysis of endometrial clot due to excessive production of plasminogen activator.[45] Increased local production of prostaglandin E2 and prostacyclin also may be present, thus promoting vasodilation.[46,47] At this time, however, there are no clinical tests available to diagnose these endometrial abnormalities. Other endometrial disorders, such as endometrial infection or inflammation, also may present as IMB.

Table 3
Medical management options for abnormal uterine bleeding

Combined contraceptives: oral, transdermal – cyclic or noncyclic	
Progestin-only therapies:	
Progestin-only contraceptive pills	Norethindrone
Levonorgestrel-releasing intrauterine device	(3 or 5-y product)
Medroxyprogesterone acetate (MPA)	Depo MPA 150 mg intramuscularly every 12 wk Depo-Sub Q Provera 104 mg sq every 12 wk Oral MPA 2.5–10 mg 12–14 d/mo
Megestrol acetate oral	20–40 mg 12–14 d/mo
Norethindrone acetate oral	2.5–5.0 mg 12–14 d/mo
Micronized progesterone	Oral 200–400 mg 12–14 d/mo
Adjuvant medical agents:	
Tranexamic acid oral	650 mg 3 times a day for 5 d
Intravenous	1–1.3 g every 6–8 h dosing during menses
Nonsteroidal anti-inflammatory agents -oral	(Alone or in combination with contraceptive medications)
Mefenamic acid	500 mg every 12 h × 4–5 d
Naproxen	275–550 mg every 12 h × 4–5 d
Ibuprofen	600–800 mg every 6–8 h × 4–5 d

Abnormalities in local inflammatory response and altered endometrial vasculogenesis or deficient molecular endometrial repair are other potential etiologies in this category. The role of an inflammatory infiltrate in the endometrium is not well understood because inflammatory cells may be present in the normal endometrium. Subclinical infection with *Chlamydia trachomatis* has been reported in association with AUB.[48] The diagnosis of AUB in this category is usually a diagnosis of exclusion.

Iatrogenic

Medical intervention including hormonal therapies or intrauterine devices can cause or contribute to AUB. Unscheduled bleeding associated with hormonal contraceptives is usually termed breakthrough bleeding (BTB) and is a major contributor to AUB of this category. Other contributors, such as bleeding disorders, infections, or anatomic abnormalities, should be excluded. Hormonal contraception associated with iatrogenic AUB (AUB-I) may result from effects on the HPO axis as wells as local effects on the endometrium. Other mechanisms contributing to AUB in the iatrogenic category include decreased circulating gonadal steroids due to patient noncompliance, medications or supplements altering steroid metabolism, impacting serotonin uptake, or cigarette smoking.[49] Progestin-only hormonal contraceptives are frequently associated with breakthrough bleeding in the first 1 to 6 months of use. HMB is a frequent occurrence in women on anticoagulant medications (warfarin, heparin, and low molecular weight heparin) due to inhibited clot formation in the endometrial vasculature. This bleeding associated with anticoagulant use, however, is placed in the AUB-C (coagulopathy) category, as it effects a systemic disorder of hemostasis.

Not Yet Classified

Several entities likely to be in the "not yet classified" (AUB-N) category include chronic endometritis, arterio-venous malformations, and myometrial hypertrophy. Future research may place these causes into separate categories or reassign them to existing categories.

In summary, appropriate categorization of women with AUB, HMB and IMB will allow clinicians to apply proven clinical therapy, communicate with other clinicians internationally, and assist future research to address etiologies and develop new therapeutic applications for these disorders.

REFERENCES

1. Fraser IS, Critchley HO, Munro MG, et al. A process designed to lead to international agreement on terminologies and definitions used to describe abnormalities of menstrual bleeding. Fertil Steril 2007;87(3):466–76.
2. Fraser IS, Critchley HO, Munro MG, et al. Can we achieve international agreement on terminologies and definitions used to describe abnormalities of menstrual bleeding? Hum Reprod 2007;22(3):635.
3. Treloar AE, Boynton RE, Behn BG, et al. Variation of the human menstrual cycle through reproductive life. Int J Fertil 1967;12:77–126.
4. Hallberg L, Hogdahl AM, Nilsson L, et al. Menstrual blood loss; a population study. Acta Obstet Gynecol Scand 1966;45:320–51.
5. Munro MG, Critchley HO, Broder MS, et al. FIGO classification system (PALM-COEIN) for causes of abnormal uterine bleeding in nongravid women of reproductive age. Int J Gynaecol Obstet 2011;113:3–13.
6. Kerner H, Lichtig C. Mullerian adenosarcoma presenting as cervical polyps: a report of seven cases and review of the literature. Obstet Gynecol 1993;81:655.

7. Lee SC, Kaunitz AM, Sanchez-Ramos L, et al. The oncogenic potential of endometrial polyps: a systematic review and metaanalysis. Obstet Gynecol 2010;116: 1197.

8. Kuokkanen S, Pal L. Steroid hormone receptor profile of premenopausal endometrial polyps. Reprod Sci 2010;17:377.

9. Jovanovic AS, Boynton KA, Mutter GL. Uteri of women with endometrial cancer contain a histopathological spectrum of monoclonal putative precancers, some with microsatellite instability. Cancer Res 1996;56:1917.

10. Pal K, Niklaus AL, Kim M, et al. Heterogeneity in endometrial expression of aromatase in polyp-bearing uteri. Hum Reprod 2008;23:80.

11. Maia H Jr, Pimentel K, Silva TM, et al. Aromatase and cyclooxygenase-2 expression in endometrial polyps during the menstrual cycle. Gynecol Endocrinol 2006; 22:219.

12. Dal Cin P, Vanni R, Marras S, et al. Four cytogenetic subgroups can be identified in endometrial polyps. Cancer Res 1995;55:1565.

13. Nogueira AA, Sant'Ana de Almeida EC, Poli Neto OB, et al. Immunohistochemical expression of p63 in endometrial polyps: evidence that a basal cell immunophenotype is maintained. Menopause 2006;13:826.

14. Beal HN, Stone J, Beckman MJ, et al. Endometrial cells identified in cervical cytology in women > or = 40 years of age: criteria for appropriate endometrial evaluation. Am J Obstet Gynecol 2007;196:568.e1.

15. DeWaay DJ, Syrop CH, Nygaard IE, et al. Natural history of uterine polyps and leiomyomata. Obstet Gynecol 2002;100:3.

16. Baiocchi G, Manci N, Pazzaglia M, et al. Malignancy in endometrial polyps: a 12 year experience. AmJ Obstet Gynecol 2009;115:206.

17. Gardner FJ, Konje JC, Bell SC, et al. Prevention of Tamoxifen induced endometrial polyps using a levonorgestrel releasing system: long term followup of a randomized controlled trial. Obstet Gynecol 2013;121:943.

18. Templeman C, Marshall SF, Ursin G, et al. Adenomyosis and endometriosis in the California Teachers Study. Fertil Steril 2008;90:415.

19. Taran FA, Weaver AL, Coddngton CC, et al. Understanding adenomyosis: a case control study. Fertil Steril 2010;94:1223.

20. Sheng J, Zhang WY, Zhang JP, et al. The LNG-IUS study on adenomyosis: a 3-year follow-up study on the efficacy and side effects of the use of levonorgestrel intrauterine system for the treatment of dysmenorrhea associated with adenomyosis. Contraception 2009;74:412.

21. Wang PH, Liu WM, Fuh JL, et al. Comparison of surgery alone and combined surgical-medical treatment in the management of symptomatic uterine adenomyoma. Fertil Steril 2009;92:876.

22. Nijenhuis RJ, Smeets AJ, Morpurgo M, et al. Uterine artery embolization for symptomatic adenomyosis with polyzene F-coated hydrogel microspheres: three-year clinical follow-up using UFS-QOL questionnaire. Cardiovasc Intervent Radiol 2015;38:65.

23. Zhou M, Chen JY, Tang LD, et al. Ultrasound-guided high-intensity focused ultrasound ablation for adenomyosis: the experience of a single center. Fertil Steril 2011;95:900.

24. Day Baird D, Drunson DB, Hill MC, et al. High cumulative incidence of uterine leiomyoma in black and white women: ultrasound evidence. Am J Obstet Gynecol 2003;188(1):100–7.

25. Stewart EA. Uterine fibroids. Lancet 2001;357:293.

26. Puri K, Famuyide AO, Erwin PJ, et al. Submucosal fibroids and the relation to heavy menstrual bleeding and anemia. Am J Obstet Gynecol 2014;210:38.e1.

27. Stewart EA, Nowak RA. Leiomyoma-related bleeding: a classic hypothesis updated for the molecular era. Hum Reprod Update 1996;2:295.

28. Stewart EA, Morton CC. The genetics of uterine leiomyomata: what clinicians need to know. Obstet Gynecol 2006;107:917.

29. Van Voorhis BJ, Romitti PA, Jones MP. Family history as a risk factor for development of uterine leiomyomas. Results of a pilot study. J Reprod Med 2002;47:663.

30. Grigorieva V, Chen-Mok M, Tarasova M, et al. Use of a levonorgestrel-releasing intrauterine system to treat bleeding related to uterine leiomyomas. Fertil Steril 2003;79:1194.

31. Starczewski A, Iwanicki M. Intrauterine therapy with Levonorgestrel releasing IUD of women with hypermenorrhea secondary to uterine fibroids. Ginekol Pol 2000; 71:1221 [in Polish].

32. Gupta JK, Sinha AS, Lumsden MA, et al. Uterine artery embolization for symptomatic uterine fibroids. Cochrane Database Syst Rev 2012;(5):CD005073.

33. Van der Kooij SM, Bipat S, Hehenkamp WJ, et al. Uterine artery embolization versus surgery in the treatment of symptomatic fibroids: a systematic review and metaanalysis. Am J Obstet Gynecol 2011;205:317.e1.

34. Spies JB, Bruno J, Czeyda-Pommersheim F, et al. Long-term outcome of uterine artery embolization of leiomyomata. Obstet Gynecol 2005;106:933.

35. Hesley GK, Gorny KR, Henrichsen TL, et al. A clinical review of focused ultrasound ablation with magnetic resonance guidance: an option for treating uterine fibroids. Ultrasound Q 2008;24:131.

36. Available at: http://www.nice.org.uk/nicemedia/live/11349/57237/57237.pdf. Accessed August 23, 2016.

37. Vilos GA, Allaire C, Laberge PY, et al. The management of uterine leiomyomas. J Obstet Gynaecol Can 2015;37:157.

38. Marret H, Fritel X, Ouldamer L, et al. Therapeutic management of uterine fibroid tumors: updated French guidelines. Eur J Obstet Gynecol Reprod Biol 2012;165: 156.

39. Pérez-Lopez FR, Ornat L, Ceausu I, et al. EMAS position statement management of uterine fibroids. Maturitas 2014;79:106.

40. Baak JP, Mutter GL, Robboy S, et al. The molecular genetics and morphometry-based endometrial intraepithelial neoplasia classification system predicts disease progression in endometrial hyperplasia more accurately then the 1994 World Health Organization classification system. Cancer 2005;103:2304.

41. Reed SD, Newton KM, Clinton WL, et al. Incidence of endometrial hyperplasia. Am J Obstet Gynecol 2009;6:678.e1-6.

42. Suh-Burgmann E, Hung YY, Armstrong MA. Complex atypical endometrial hyperplasia: the risk of unrecognized adenocarcinoma and value of preoperative dilatation and curettage. Obstet Gynecol 2009;114:523.

43. Reed SD, Voigt LF, Newton KM, et al. Progestin therapy of complex endometrial hyperplasia with and without atypia. Obstet Gynecol 2009;113:655.

44. Shankar M, Lee CA, Sabin CA, et al. von Willebrand disease in women with menorrhagia: a systematic review. BJOG 2004;111(7):734–40.

45. Smith SK, Abel MH, Kelly RW, et al. Prostaglandin synthesis in the endometrium of women with ovular dysfunctional uterine bleeding. Br J Obstet Gynaecol 1981; 88(4):434–42.

46. Gleeson NC. Cyclic changes in endometrial tissue plasminogen activator and plasminogen activator inhibitor type 1 in women with normal menstruation and essential menorrhagia. Am J Obstet Gynecol 1994;171(1):178–83.
47. Smith SK, Abel MH, Kelly RW, et al. A role for prostacyclin (PGi2) in excessive menstrual bleeding. Lancet 1981;1(8219):522–4.
48. Toth M, Patton DL, Esquenazi B, et al. Association between *Chlamydia trachomatis* and abnormal uterine bleeding. Am J Reprod Immunol 2007;57(5):361–6.
49. Rosenberg MJ, Waugh MS, Stevens CM. Smoking and cycle control among oral contraceptive users. Am J Obstet Gynecol 1996;174(2):628–32.

Recognition and Therapeutic Options for Malignancy of the Cervix and Uterus

Elizabeth R. Burton, MD[a],*, Joel I. Sorosky, MD[b]

KEYWORDS

- Cervical and endometrial cancer • Prevention • Risk factors • Genetics • Screening
- Treatment

KEY POINTS

- The recommendations of the American Board of Internal Medicine's Choosing Wisely campaign as they pertain to cervical and endometrial cancer are presented.
- An update on the current epidemiology and a review of the risk factors of cervical and endometrial cancers are discussed.
- Cervical cancer prevention with a focus on HPV vaccination and cervical cancer screening is reviewed, emphasizing the new focus of less frequent intervention in an effort to maintain high rates of early detection of disease while decreasing unnecessary and anxiety-provoking colposcopies, biopsies, and excisional procedures.
- The replacement of traditional endometrial hyperplasia terminology with more relevant clinical categories, with an emphasis on the introduction of endometrial intraepithelial neoplasia (EIN) is presented.
- Fertility-sparing options in the management of early cervical and endometrial cancers are reviewed.

Disclosure Statement: The authors have nothing to disclose.
[a] Division of Gynecologic Oncology, Department of Obstetrics and Gynecology, Hanjani Institute of Gynecologic Oncology, Abington Hospital, Jefferson Health, The Sidney Kimmel Medical College, Thomas Jefferson University, 1200 Old York Road, 1 Weidner Building, Abington, PA 19001, USA; [b] Department of Obstetrics and Gynecology, Hanjani Institute of Gynecologic Oncology, Abington Hospital, Jefferson Health, The Sidney Kimmel Medical College, Thomas Jefferson University, 1200 Old York Road, 1 Weidner Building, Abington, PA 19001, USA
* Corresponding author.
E-mail address: elizabeth.burton@jefferson.edu

Obstet Gynecol Clin N Am 44 (2017) 195–206
http://dx.doi.org/10.1016/j.ogc.2017.02.009
0889-8545/17/© 2017 Elsevier Inc. All rights reserved.

obgyn.theclinics.com

CERVICAL CANCER
Epidemiology/Risk Factors

The American Cancer Society estimated that there would be 12,990 new cases of invasive cervical cancer diagnosed in 2016. It was estimated that 4120 women would die from cervical cancer.[1] Cervical cancer is most common in Hispanics, African Americans, and those women of lower socioeconomic classes. These women have a high age-adjusted death rate. Risk factors for cervical cancer are high-risk human papillomavirus (HPV), smoking, early sexual activity, increased number of partners, increased parity, family history, use of oral contraceptives, immunosuppression, and diethylstilbestrol exposure.

Squamous cell carcinoma comprises most cervical cancer cases (approximately 80%–85%); however, the percentage of adenocarcinoma is rising because screening is better identifying dysplastic squamous lesions. Cervical cancer, especially at an early stage, is usually asymptomatic. Presenting symptoms may include postcoital bleeding and/or other irregular vaginal bleeding. Diagnosis is made with tissue biopsy, not pap test. Radiation and chemotherapy is generally the treatment. In early stage cervical cancer up to and including stage IB1, surgery can equal the results of radiation therapy and avoid the risks of destroying ovarian function. Fertility-sparing options do exist for properly chosen women with early stage disease.

Cervical Cancer Prevention and Human Papillomavirus Vaccine

HPV-16 and -18 are implicated in most cases of cervical cancer. Along with the woman's immune system and environmental factors, such as cigarette smoking, these two high-risk HPV genotypes (16 and 18) account for 55% to 60% and 10% to 15%, respectively, of cervical cancer cases worldwide. An additional approximately 12 oncogenic HPV genotypes comprise the remainder of the cervical cancer cases.[2] HPV is associated with anogenital cancers other than just cervical cancer: vaginal, vulvar, penile, and anal. It is also associated with oropharyngeal cancer, and genital warts.

The Centers for Disease Control and Prevention and the American College of Obstetricians and Gynecologists recommend routine HPV vaccination for females ages 9 to 26 to prevent preinvasive and invasive disease. Preliminary data from Australia and Canada demonstrate a reduction of preinvasive disease in vaccinated women.[2] There are three different vaccines available in the United States: a bivalent vaccine, which covers HPV-16 and HPV-18; a quadrivalent vaccine, which covers HPV-6 and HPV-11 in addition to HPV-16 and HPV-18; and a nine-valent vaccine, which covers an additional five high-risk HPV genotypes.[3] All three vaccines are administered in a three-dose series with a schedule of 0, 1 to 2, and 6 months. Current studies are monitoring the durability of the immune response. There is no current recommendation for a booster vaccine. The series does not need to be restarted if there is a delay in a second or third dose. A local injection reaction of swelling and edema is common, especially with the nine-valent vaccine. Providers should counsel parents and patients to expect, and not be alarmed by, discomfort and a local site reaction after the vaccination. There have been no significant adverse reactions to the HPV vaccine after greater than 60 million administered doses. Vaccine administration during pregnancy should be avoided, with doses of a series being delayed until completion of pregnancy and breastfeeding. Inadvertent administration of vaccine during pregnancy is not thought to cause harm based on data available at this time.[3]

The Advisory Committee on Immunization Practices recommends the nine-valent HPV vaccine, approved by the US Food and Drug Administration in December 2014 for girls and boys aged 11 to 12 years. Catch-up vaccination is recommended through age 26 for those males and females not vaccinated in the target age range.[3] HPV vaccination of girls at an earlier age (9–14 years vs 15–26 years) results in higher antibody levels.[3] It is unclear if this increased immune response correlates with vaccine efficacy. Earlier vaccination is preferred because vaccines are most effective when given before the onset of sexual activity, therefore before exposure to HPV. Vaccination is still indicated even if follows the onset of sexual activity, because it is unlikely a woman has been exposed to all HPV genotypes in the vaccine. There is no indication for HPV testing before vaccination.[3]

Australia has a population-based vaccination program with high adherence. A decrease in high-grade cervical abnormalities was noted within 3 years of program initiation.[2] The United States has seen low vaccination rates. Only 50% of girls aged 13 to 17 years have received at least one vaccine. Only 33% of girls in the recommended age group have received all three vaccines.[3] In June 2016, the Society of Gynecologic Oncology submitted seven recommendations to Vice President Joe Biden's National Cancer Moonshot initiative. One of the recommendations was for school-based HPV vaccination in an effort to improve vaccination rates and therefore decrease incidence of cervical dysplasia and cancer.

Along with a recommendation to mothers to vaccinate boys and girls, obstetrics and gynecology health care providers should counsel young women on the benefits of protected sexual intercourse. Providers should advise women to cease smoking. They should counsel women who are immunocompromised of their higher risk for persistent HPV infection. Providers should encourage all women to present for routine screening. Immunocompromised women should follow a stricter screening schedule depending on the clinical situation.

Cervical Cancer Screening

HPV infection is usually transient, with spontaneous regression. The lifetime risk of HPV infection is greater than 80%. In one study, HPV infection occurred at least once over a 3-year period in 60% of young women. In young women, especially those younger than 21 years of age, an effective immune response results in the resolution of an HPV infection in an average of 8 months after exposure. A total of 85% to 90% of young women clear the virus or have undetectable viral load in an average of 8 to 24 months. The few HPV infections that are persistent at 1 to 2 years are more likely to lead to high-grade cervical dysplasia and/or cancer. Cervical dysplasia usually resolves with the resolution of the virus, whereas persistent viral infection results in persistent dysplasia.[4]

Newly acquired HPV infection has the same low chance of persistence in women older than age 30. However, HPV infection in women older than age 30 is more likely to reflect persistent infection, and therefore more likely associated with high-grade dysplasia. Untreated high-grade cervical intraepithelial neoplasia-3 progresses to cervical cancer in 30% of the cases at 30 years.[2] This means 70% do not progress into cancer and allows the opportunity for conservative management in selective cases where childbearing has not yet been completed. Close follow-up with colposcopy every 6 months is required. Progression of disease in most HPV-related types of cervical neoplasia is slow. Because the progression likely takes more than 8 to 10 years, less frequent screening is not unreasonable.

Screening programs in the United States have led to decrease in incidence of cervical cancer by more than 50% in the past 30 years. In 1975, the rate of cervical cancer was 14.8 per 100,000 women. By 2011, the rate decreased to 6.7 per 100,000 women.[2] Mortality has similarly decreased. Most women diagnosed with cervical cancer either never had cervical cancer testing or have not been screened within 5 years of diagnosis. It is predicted that it will take 20 years after widespread vaccination before there is a significant reduction in the incident of cervical cancer cases. Screening recommendations apply regardless of HPV vaccination status.

Indications for HPV testing, to test for the presence of high-risk HPV, are changing as more knowledge is attained. Currently, indications include the following[2]:

- Determination of the need for colposcopy in women with a cytology result of atypical squamous cell of undetermined significance ("reflex testing").
- Use as an adjunct to cytology for cervical cancer screening in women aged 30 to 65 years and older ("cotesting").
- One HPV test was approved by the Food and Drug Administration in 2014 for primary cervical cancer screening in women 25 years and older.

Indications for HPV genotyping are currently limited to negative pap test results (cytology) but positive high-risk HPV test results in women aged 30 to 65 years who are undergoing cotesting. If the HPV genotyping determines infection is with HPV-16 or -18, colposcopy is recommended.[2] Otherwise, the recommendation is repeat cotesting in 1 year.

The goal of current screening efforts is to balance the benefits of screening with the risks, which include costly, unnecessary, and anxiety-provoking colposcopies, biopsies, and excisional procedures. These additional procedures also potentially negatively affect reproductive outcomes. One study found a significant increase in rates of preterm birth among women previously treated with excisional procedures for neoplasia. The recent revisions to the screening guidelines have incorporated the powerful negative predictive value of HPV testing and lengthening screening intervals (**Box 1**). Liquid-based and conventional methods of cervical cytology collection are acceptable for screening.

Box 1
Screening recommendations of the American Cancer Society, the American Society for Colposcopy and Cervical Pathology, and the American Society for Clinical Pathology

- Women younger than 21 years: No screening.

- Women aged 21 to 29 years: Cytology alone every 3 years.

- Women aged 30 to 65 years: HPV and cytology cotesting every 5 years (preferred); cytology alone every 3 years (acceptable). Recent change: HPV testing alone using Food and Drug Administration–approved HPV test.

- Women older than 65 years: No screening is necessary after adequate negative prior screening results. Twenty years of routine screening is required for any women with a history of cervical intraepithelial neoplasia-2 or -3, or adenocarcinoma in situ. This recommendation does not change even in the event of a new sexual partner because cervical cancer occurs a median of 15 to 25 years after HPV infection.

- Women who underwent total hysterectomy: No screening is necessary in women without a cervix and no history of cervical intraepithelial neoplasia-2 or -3, or adenocarcinoma in situ in the past 20 years.

- Women vaccinated against HPV: Same as unvaccinated women.

Adapted from Committee on Practice Bulletins-Gynecology. Cervical cancer screening and prevention. Practice Bulletin No. 168. American College of Obstetricians and Gynecologists. Obstet Gynecol 2016; 128: e111–30.

Endocervical curettage is indicated in women with atypical squamous cells of undetermined significance or low-grade squamous intraepithelial lesion cervical cytology results when no lesion is identified on colposcopy, when the colposcopic examination is unsatisfactory, and in women with previous excision or ablation of the transformation zone. Additionally, in women with atypical squamous cells that cannot rule out high-grade (high-grade intraepithelial lesion), atypical glandular cells, or adenocarcinoma in situ, endocervical curettage should be considered unless an excisional procedure is planned. If an excisional procedure is planned, endocervical curettage may be performed at the time of the procedure to assess completeness of the procedure.[4] These screening recommendations are not meant for women with cervical cancer, human immunodeficiency virus infection, immunosuppression for any reason, or exposure to diethylstilbestrol in utero, and may not apply to women with solid organ transplants.

Cervical Cancer Fertility-Sparing Treatment

The treatment of early stage cervical cancer is surgical. Locally advanced cervical cancer treatment is radiation therapy and sensitizing chemotherapy. Neither standard surgery, nor chemotherapy/radiation therapy spare the option of future childbearing for women who are of childbearing age. There are fertility-sparing surgical options for women of childbearing age with early stage cervical cancers. Fertility-sparing approaches are not standard, but they are acceptable in appropriate patients and allow for fertility with plan for completion surgery once the postpartum period is complete.

Cervical cancer is the most common gynecologic cancer diagnosed during pregnancy. Breast cancer is the most common cancer diagnosed during pregnancy. Most women with a new diagnosis of cervical cancer are still of childbearing age, because most cases occur in women in their fourth or fifth decade of life (30s and 40s). Fertility-sparing option for stage IA1 cervical cancer is a cold knife cone. For stage IA2 cervical cancer, a radical trachelectomy with lymphadenectomy is appropriate in select women (**Box 2**).

The Choosing Wisely Campaign's recommendations and highlights in regards to cervical cancer are discussed later along with those recommendations regarding endometrial cancer.[5–13]

ENDOMETRIAL CANCER
Epidemiology/Risk Factors

Endometrial cancer is the most common gynecologic malignancy in the United States. Women in the United States have a 3% lifetime risk of developing endometrial cancer. The National Cancer Institute Surveillance, Epidemiology, and End Results Program database estimated there would be 60,050 new cases of endometrial cancer in 2016, with an estimated 10,470 deaths from endometrial cancer in 2016.[14] Endometrial cancer is the fourth leading cause of cancer, and the seventh leading cause of cancer death. Endometrial cancer is more common in white women, but black women have a higher mortality from the disease. It is uncertain why this disparity exists.[1]

Risk factors are estrogen exposure, tamoxifen use, estrogen-producing tumors, and prior pelvic radiation therapy. Women with body mass index greater than 30 have two to three times the risk of developing endometrial cancer. Women with body mass index greater than 40 have significantly shorter survival and experienced more deaths unrelated to their endometrial cancer diagnosis when compared with nonobese women.[15] Oral contraceptive use and smoking reduce risk of developing endometrial cancer.

Box 2
International Federation of Obstetricians and Gynecologists clinical stages of cervical cancer, revised 2009

0. Carcinoma in situ, cervical intraepithelial lesion-3

I. Carcinoma is strictly confined to cervix (extension to corpus should be disregarded)
   IA. Microscopic lesion, invasion is limited to measured stromal invasion with a maximum depth of 5 mm and no wider than 7 mm
      IA1. Measured invasion of stroma no greater than 3 mm in depth and no wider than 7 mm
      IA2. Measured invasion of stroma greater than 3 mm and no greater than 5 mm in depth and no wider than 7 mm
   IB. Clinical lesions confined to the cervix or preclinical lesions greater than IA
      IB1. Clinical lesions no greater than 4 cm in size
      IB2. Clinical lesions greater than 4 cm in size

II. Carcinoma extends beyond cervix but has not extended to pelvic side wall; it involves vagina, but not as far as the lower third

III. Carcinoma has extended to the pelvic wall; on rectal examination there is no cancer-free space between tumor and pelvic wall; tumor involves lower third of vagina; all cases with hydronephrosis or nonfunctioning kidney should be included, unless they are known to be due to another cause

IV. Carcinoma has extended beyond true pelvis or has clinically involved mucosa of bladder or rectum
   IVA. Spread of growth to adjacent pelvic organs
   IVB. Spread to distant organs

Adapted from Pecorelli S. Revised FIGO staging for carcinoma of the vulva, cervix, and endometrium. Int J Gynaecol Obstet 2009;105(2):104; with permission.

Presentation, Diagnosis, and Treatment

The most common presenting symptom is menometrorrhagia in a premenopausal woman, and postmenopausal bleeding in a postmenopausal woman. Diagnosis is made with endometrial sampling in the office with an endometrial biopsy, or with dilation and curettage with or without hysteroscopic assistance. The pap test has no role in diagnosis, but endometrial cells in a postmenopausal woman confers a 3% to 5% risk of endometrial cancer and needs further evaluation. Atypical glandular cells on pap also requires further evaluation with endometrial sampling in women older than 35 or in younger women with risk factors for endometrial cancer.

A minimally invasive technique is now the standard surgical approach. The Gynecologic Oncology Group demonstrated in the LAP2 study that laparoscopic surgical staging for endometrial cancer is safe and feasible, resulting in fewer complications and in shorter hospital stays. A follow-up study demonstrated almost identical 5-year survival at 89.8% for early stage disease.[15] When laparoscopy has been compared with robotic surgery for endometrial cancer, outcomes are similar with the exception of lower blood loss, but longer operative times for the robotic cases.

Type I disease is the most common, and is most commonly endometrioid type histology. These tumors may have microsatellite instability and mutations in PTEN, PIK3CA, K-ras, and CTNNBI.[15] Type II disease is less common, at approximately 10% of the endometrial cancer cases. Type II disease is usually high grade, is of serous or clear cell histology, and occurs in older and more commonly in black women. Approximately 10% to 30% of these tumors exhibit p53 mutations.[15] Treatment of type I (estrogen dependent) and type II (estrogen independent) endometrial cancer is the same with total hysterectomy and bilateral salpingo-oophorectomy the gold standard. The role of lymph node assessment and postoperative adjuvant radiation therapy remain controversial.

Preoperative imaging chest radiograph is appropriate. Use of CA125 preoperatively in an effort to predict extrauterine disease is controversial. An elevated CA125 has been reported to be the single most significant predictor of extrauterine disease.[15]

Gynecologic oncologists are incorporating sentinel lymph node evaluation at the time of surgery. Although some surgeons are incorporating injection of isosulphan blue dye into the uterine cervix before laparotomy or standard laparoscopy, most are incorporating sentinel lymph node evaluation at the time of robotic hysterectomy. An accepted approach is injection of indocyanine green dye at 3 and 9 o'clock on the face of the cervix. Florescence technology available on the robotic platform allows for identification of sentinel lymph nodes.

Fertility-sparing options do exist for properly chosen women with early stage disease. Hormonal therapy and/or primary radiation therapy are options for women who are medically inoperable.

Endometrial Intraepithelial Neoplasia

Endometrial hyperplasia is a known precursor to endometrial adenocarcinoma, endometrioid type (or type I). In 1994, the World Health Organization proposed the categories of endometrial hyperplasia as simple hyperplasia without atypia, complex hyperplasia without atypia, simple hyperplasia with atypia, and complex hyperplasia with atypia.[16]

The American College of Obstetrics and Gynecology has now recommended new criteria that have more clinical relevance: benign, premalignant, and malignant.[16] This endometrial intraepithelial neoplasia (EIN) schema is replacing 1994 World Health Organization categories for precancer of endometrium. Specifically, the category of EIN now replaces that previously known as endometrial complex atypical hyperplasia, which confers a 40% risk of malignancy in the hysterectomy specimen (**Box 3**).

Gynecologists are encouraged to consider evaluation of the endometrial cavity with dilation and curettage with hysteroscopy to differentiate between the true premalignant EIN and endometrial carcinoma. Hysteroscopy is better than curettage at detecting polyps, submucosal leiomyomas, and focal areas of disease in the endometrial cavity. Although hysteroscopy may potentially disseminate tumor from the endometrial cavity into the peritoneal cavity, there is no evidence that use of hysteroscopy to diagnose endometrial cancer alters prognosis of the disease.

Preoperative planning for a diagnosis of endometrial cancer should include involvement by gynecologic oncology because intraoperative findings may dictate surgical

---

Box 3
Diagnostic criteria for endometrial intraepithelial neoplasia

- Benign endometrial hyperplasia: diffuse topography caused by prolonged estrogen effect. Treatment: hormonal therapy for symptomatic relief.

- Endometrial intraepithelial neoplasia: focal progressing to diffuse topography, which is considered precancerous. Treatment: hormonal therapy or surgery.

- Endometrial adenocarcinoma: focal progressing to diffuse topography, which is considered malignant. Treatment: surgery, stage based.

Adapted from Committee on Gynecologic Practice, Society of Gynecologic Oncology. The American College of Obstetricians and Gynecologists committee opinion no. 631. Endometrial intraepithelial neoplasia. Obstet Gynecol 2015;125(5):1273.

staging. Studies have demonstrated that primary management by gynecologic oncology resulted in efficient use of health care resources and minimized morbidity. Additionally, a known preoperative diagnosis of endometrial cancer would allow counseling and preparation of the woman for the possibility of a need for genetic counseling, postoperative treatment with chemotherapy, and/or radiation therapy.

Treatment options for EIN and endometrial cancer remain the same with total hysterectomy being the gold standard for definitive diagnosis and treatment. The use of supracervical hysterectomy, morcellation, and endometrial ablation are never acceptable options for the treatment of EIN.[16]

Fertility-sparing options include systemic or local progesterone therapy with a goal of reversal of premalignancy or low-grade malignancy. Notably, there is neither a consensus nor are there clear guidelines regarding the dose, scheduling, length of treatment, and posttreatment surveillance for premalignant endometrial disease.[15,16] Of note, the underlying cause of the estrogenic environment (estrogen as mitogen) remains unchanged in most cases, thus progesterone treatment may only delay an inevitable development of EIN to cancer.

Medical management also remains an appropriate effort to control disease in patients with medical comorbidities too significant to tolerate general anesthesia and surgical intervention.

To prevent development and recurrence of endometrial precancer and/or cancer, gynecologists should recommend continued efforts of weight loss through diet, exercise, and/or bariatric surgery.

Endometrial Cancer Genetics

Lynch syndrome, also known as hereditary nonpolyposis colorectal cancer, is an autosomal-dominant mutation of one of four most commonly affected mismatch repair genes. The most common genes associated with Lynch syndrome are MLH1 MSH2, MSH6, and PMS2. Defects in these mismatch repair genes lead to a phenomenon called microsatellite instability, which then leads to development of malignancy.

In women with Lynch syndrome, the most frequent cancers noted are colorectal, endometrial, and ovarian. Three percent of all endometrial cancer cases are related to Lynch syndrome. Lynch syndrome accounts for the most heritable cases of endometrial and colorectal malignancies.[17] These Lynch syndrome–related cancers emerge 10 to 15 years earlier than in sporadic cases. Nearly 10% of endometrial cancers diagnosed before age 50 are associated with Lynch syndrome.[17] The American College of Obstetrics and Gynecologists along with the Society of Gynecologic Oncology recommends universal screening for Lynch syndrome for all women with newly diagnosed endometrial cancers.

In one retrospective study of women with Lynch syndrome who developed gynecologic and gastrointestinal malignancies, the presenting cancer was gynecologic in greater than 50% of the women.[17] This validates universal screening of all endometrial cancers because it may affect surveillance for other malignancies if a patient tests positive for a gene mutation. According to the American College of Obstetrics and Gynecologists and the Society of Gynecologic Oncology, universal screening provides the most sensitive approach for accurate detection of Lynch syndrome cases with the lowest risk of false negatives. Universal screening is not very specific, but screening based on clinical characteristics alone may miss up to 30% of Lynch syndrome–associated endometrial and colorectal cancers.[17] Screening involves testing tumor tissue immunohistochemically labeled for mismatch repair system proteins. If the immunohistochemical testing is suggestive of a mutation, then germline testing is performed (**Box 4**).

> **Box 4**
> **Recommendations for patients with Lynch syndrome**
>
> - Screening colonoscopies starting at age 20 to 25, or 2 to 5 years before earliest familial diagnosis of cancer.
> - Endometrial biopsies every 1 to 2 years beginning at age 30 to 35 years.
> - Chemoprevention with oral contraceptive pills/progestin-based therapy.
> - Ultrasounds to screen for ovarian cancer.
> - To consider prophylactic hysterectomy and bilateral salpingo-oophorectomy at the completion of childbearing.
>
> *Adapted from* Committee on Practice Bulletins-Gynecology, Society of Gynecologic Oncology. ACOG practice bulletin no. 147: Lynch syndrome. Obstet Gynecol 2014;124(5):1042–54.

The Society of Gynecologic Oncology position statement from October 2014 regarding genetic testing for gynecologic cancer is as follows: "All women diagnosed with endometrial cancer should be assessed for Lynch Syndrome. In addition, women with a family history of endometrial cancer and colon cancer should pursue genetic counseling regardless of whether they have been diagnosed with cancer." In June 2013, the US Supreme Court ruled in a unanimous decision to invalidate human gene patents. This leveling of the playing field allowed for the rapid expansion and greater affordability of genetic testing (**Box 5**).

Endometrial Cancer Fertility-Sparing Treatment

The mean age for endometrial adenocarcinoma is 61 years, with most cases diagnosed between the ages of 50 and 60 years. However, 20% of women are diagnosed before menopause and approximately 5% of women have a diagnosis before age 40.[15] For this 5% and those with additional patients with EIN, fertility-sparing options are inevitably part of the initial conversation.

The gold standard treatment of endometrial cancer is total hysterectomy with bilateral salpingo-oophorectomy. Postoperative chemotherapy with or without radiation therapy depends on extent and distribution of disease noted at time of surgery.

The gold standard of surgery does not allow for future fertility. There are fertility-sparing surgical and medical options for women of childbearing age with clinical early stage, low-grade endometrial cancers. Fertility-sparing approaches are controversial without clear guidelines from cooperative societies.

MRI should be obtained before offering fertility-sparing options in an effort to evaluate for myometrial invasion. Myometrial invasion is a contraindication to

> **Box 5**
> **Recommendations for unaffected patients who should be offered genetic testing**
>
> - First-degree relative less than 60 years old with endometrial or colorectal cancer.
> - Multiple generations of family members with Lynch syndrome–associated cancers.
> - Remote relative in the family where multiple family members had early hysterectomies/oophorectomy, and/or family with a small number of female relatives, and/or many early deaths.
>
> *Adapted from* Committee on Practice Bulletins-Gynecology, Society of Gynecologic Oncology. ACOG practice bulletin no. 147: Lynch syndrome. Obstet Gynecol 2014;124(5):1042–54.

conservative, fertility-sparing management. The limitations of MRI should be noted. Although MRI has been demonstrated to have negative predictive value, it does not have the sensitivity, positive predictive value, or the accuracy to make confident clinical decisions.[15] MRI is far better than computed tomography or any other imaging modality to evaluate the endomyometrial junction.

Fertility-sparing options begin with dilation and curettage with hysteroscopy in an effort to reduce the tumor burden of the endometrial lining. Either oral megestrol acetate, 80 mg twice daily, or a levonorgestrel intrauterine device to administer local progesterone to endometrial lining and uterine cavity, is an accepted medical management.

Recurrence rates are high. In one study, complete response was found in 55% of endometrial carcinomas and 82% of atypical endometrial hyperplasia. Although there are seven normal deliveries among the 45 study candidates, there was a 47% recurrence rate between 7 and 36 months, and one woman died of a synchronous ovarian cancer.[15]

An accepted approach to monitor the uterine cavity is with endometrial biopsy or dilation and curettage every 3 to 6 months. Fertility therapy must follow resolution of the endometrial pathology.[15] Definitive management is total hysterectomy at the completion of child-bearing. A bilateral salpingo-oophorectomy is also recommended. Exceptions to bilateral salpingo-oophorectomy can occur in younger women.

In obese women, endogenous estrogen from peripheral conversion of androstenedione into estrone can result in continued unopposed proliferation of the endometrial lining. Anovulation results in continuous unopposed estrogen stimulation because there is no corpus luteum to produce progesterone. Nulliparity is associated with a two- to three-fold increased incidence of disease.[15] Women seeking fertility-sparing management for EIN or grade 1 endometrial cancer should be encouraged to pursue multibehavioral lifestyle changes to complement medical and surgical efforts to reverse the disease process. Recent studies suggest that bariatric surgery may decrease these risks, but additional validation is required (**Box 6**).

Box 6
International Federation of Gynecology and Obstetrics Surgical Staging System for Endometrial Cancer, revised 2009

I. Tumor confined to the corpus uteri
  IA. No or less than half myometrial invasion
  IB. Invasion equal to or more than half of the myometrium

II. Tumor invades cervical stroma, but does not extend beyond the uterus

III. Local and/or regional spread of tumor
  IIIA. Tumor invades the serosa of the corpus uteri and/or adnexae
  IIIB. Vaginal and/or parametrial involvement
  IIIC. Metastases to pelvic and/or para-aortic lymph nodes
    IIIC1. Positive pelvic nodes
    IIIC2. Positive paraaortic lymph nodes with or without positive pelvic lymph nodes

IV. Tumor invades bladder and/or bowel mucosa, and/or distant metastases
  IVA. Tumor invasion of bladder and/or bowel mucosa
  IVB. Distant metastases, including intra-abdominal metastases and/or inguinal lymph nodes

Adapted from Pecorelli S. Revised FIGO staging for carcinoma of the vulva, cervix, and endometrium. Int J Gynaecol Obstet 2009;105(2):104; with permission.

Choosing Wisely Campaign Highlights

The American Board of Internal Medicine launched Choosing Wisely in 2012 as an effort to control the use of "wasteful or unnecessary medical tests, treatments and procedures" in this country.[5] The American Board of Internal Medicine features more than 70 different subspecialties, highlighting areas where evidence-based medicine has demonstrated a change in practice is appropriate. In 2013, the Choosing Wisely campaign published five recommendations related to gynecologic cancers. Regarding women with a history of endometrial cancer, one recommendation is to discontinue routine pap smears for surveillance. In regards to cervical cancer and pap tests, the Choosing Wisely campaign recommends to use pap smears but to avoid colposcopy in patients treated for cervical cancer with pap tests of low-grade lesion or less. A third recommendation is to avoid routine imaging for cancer surveillance for all gynecologic malignancies.[6–13]

- Pap testing of the top of the vagina in women treated for endometrial cancer does not improve detection of local recurrence. False-positive pap tests in this group can lead to unnecessary procedures, such as colposcopy and biopsy.
- Colposcopy for low-grade abnormalities in this group does not detect recurrence unless there is a visible lesion and is not cost effective.
- Imaging in the absence of symptoms or rising tumor markers has shown low yield in detecting recurrence or impacting overall survival.

REFERENCES

1. American Cancer Society. Available at: www.cancer.org.
2. American College of Obstetrics and Gynecologists. Practice bulletin no. 157: cervical cancer screening and prevention. Obstet Gynecol 2016;127:e1–20.
3. American College of Obstetrics and Gynecologists. Committee opinion no. 641: human papillomavirus vaccination. Obstet Gynecol 2015;126:e38–43.
4. American College of Obstetrics and Gynecologists. Practice bulletin no. 140: management of abnormal cervical cancer screening test results and cervical cancer precursors. Obstet Gynecol 2013;122:1338–67.
5. Choosing Wisely, An Initiative of the ABIM Foundation. 2013. Available at: www.choosingwisely.org.
6. Salani R, Backes FJ, Fung MF, et al. Posttreatment surveillance and diagnosis of recurrence in women with gynecologic malignancies: society of gynecologic oncologists recommendations. Am J Obstet Gynecol 2011;204:466–78.
7. Salani R, Nagel CI, Drennen E, et al. Recurrence patterns and surveillance for patients with early stage endometrial cancer. Gynecol Oncol 2011;123:205–7.
8. Bristow RE, Purinton SC, Santillan A, et al. Cost-effectiveness of routine vaginal cytology for endometrial cancer surveillance. Gynecol Oncol 2006;103:709–13.
9. Sartori E, Pasinetti B, Carrara L, et al. Pattern of failure and value of follow up procedures in endometrial and cervical cancer patients. Gynecol Oncol 2007;107: S241–7.
10. Berchuck A, Anspach C, Evans AC, et al. Postsurgical surveillance of patients with FIGO stage I/II endometrial adenocarcinoma. Gynecol Oncol 1995;59:20–4.
11. Bhosale P, Peungjesada S, Wei W, et al. Clinical utility of positron emission tomography/computed tomography in the evaluation of suspected recurrent ovarian cancer in the setting of normal CA125 levels. Int J Gynecol Cancer 2010;20: 936–44.

12. Havrilesky LJ, Wong TZ, Alvarez Secord A, et al. The role of PET scanning in the detection of recurrent cervical cancer. Gynecol Oncol 2003;90:186–90.

13. Rimel BJ, Ferda A, Erwin J, et al. Cervicovaginal cytology in the detection of recurrence after cervical cancer treatment. Obstet Gynecol 2011;118:548–53.

14. National Cancer Institute, Surveillance, Epidemiology, and End Results Program. Available at: seer.cancer.gov.

15. Sorosky JI. Endometrial cancer. Obstet Gynecol 2012;120(2 Pt 1):383–97.

16. Committee on Gynecologic Practice, Society of Gynecologic Oncology. The American College of Obstetricians and Gynecologists committee opinion no. 631: endometrial intraepithelial neoplasia. Obstet Gynecol 2015;125:1272–8.

17. Committee on Practice Bulletins-Gynecology, Society of Gynecologic Oncology. ACOG practice bulletin no. 147: Lynch syndrome. Obstet Gynecol 2014;124: 1042–54.

Gestational Diabetes
Diagnosis, Classification, and Clinical Care

 CrossMark

Lynn R. Mack, MD[a], Paul G. Tomich, MD[b],*

KEYWORDS

• Gestational diabetes • Diagnosis • Classification • Clinical care

KEY POINTS

- Gestational diabetes (GDM) and newly diagnosed type 2 diabetes in pregnancy are increasingly more common in women of all races due to the obesity epidemic.
- Treating diabetes in pregnancy reduces complications.
- Optimal screening and diagnostic approaches to screen for diabetes in pregnancy are debated.
- A 75-g oral glucose tolerance test (OGTT) should be performed 6 to 12 weeks postpartum as up to 36% of women have impaired glucose tolerance postpartum.
- Women with prediabetes postpartum should be offered intensive lifestyle intervention and/or metformin to prevent progression to type 2 diabetes.

BACKGROUND

Gestational diabetes mellitus (GDM) is a condition where women without a previous diagnosis of diabetes exhibit abnormal blood glucose levels during pregnancy. In normal pregnancy pancreatic B-cell hyperplasia occurs from the stimulation of human placental lactogen and prolactin, resulting in higher insulin levels. Placental secretion of diabetogenic hormones, such as growth hormone, corticotropin-releasing hormone, placental lactogen, and progesterone, leads to increasing insulin resistance. The inability to overcome the insulin resistance of pregnancy despite B-cell hyperplasia leads to GDM. GDM in turn carries increased risks for the mother and neonate to include preeclampsia, birth weight over 4000 grams, and shoulder dystocia. Therefore, the identification and management of GDM is important.[1–3]

[a] Division of Diabetes, Endocrinology, and Metabolism, Department of Internal Medicine, 984120 Nebraska Medical Center, Omaha, NE 68198-4120, USA; [b] Division of Maternal Fetal Medicine, Department of Obstetrics and Gynecology, 983255 Nebraska Medical Center, Omaha, NE 68198-3255, USA
* Corresponding author.
E-mail address: ptomich@unmc.edu

Obstet Gynecol Clin N Am 44 (2017) 207–217
http://dx.doi.org/10.1016/j.ogc.2017.02.002
0889-8545/17/© 2017 Elsevier Inc. All rights reserved.

obgyn.theclinics.com

The prevalence of GDM in the United States is about 9% based on data from DeSisto and colleagues[4] using prevalence estimates from the Pregnancy Risk Assessment Monitoring System (PRAMS) with a range from 1% to 25% depending on ethnicity of the mother and the diagnostic criteria used for the diagnosis.[2,5] The ongoing obesity epidemic has led to more type 2 diabetes in women of childbearing age with a greater number of pregnant women with undiagnosed type 2 diabetes.[6] Therefore, it is reasonable to test women with risk factors for type 2 diabetes (**Box 1**) at their first prenatal visit with standard diagnostic criteria used in nonpregnant patients (**Box 2**).[7]

Those women identified to have diabetes in the first trimester would be classified as type 2 diabetes and not GDM, where that label is reserved for diabetes diagnosed in the second or third trimester of pregnancy and is not clearly type 1 or type 2 diabetes.

The obstetrician gynecologist caring for a pregnant woman with gestational diabetes should be knowledgeable about the maternal and fetal risks related to that diagnosis, antepartum maternal and fetal surveillance, the role of ultrasound for monitoring fetal growth and well-being, the decision-making process for the timing and route of delivery, managing blood sugars while in labor, and postpartum assessment and counseling.

In addition to routine pregnancy care, prenatal care of women who have gestational diabetes should focus on those conditions that are more common in women with glucose impairment. Short-term complications more common in women with gestational diabetes include large for gestational age infants and macrosomia, preeclampsia, polyhydramnios, stillbirth, and increased neonatal morbidity. There is not an increased risk of congenital malformations in these infants. The long-term complications associated with gestational diabetes extend beyond the postpartum period and neonatal period. These may reflect the infant's increased risk of developing childhood obesity, impaired glucose tolerance, and metabolic syndrome. For the mother, gestational diabetes is a marker for the development of type 2 diabetes later in life.

The most common adverse neonatal outcomes associated with gestational diabetes are fetal macrosomia and being large for gestational age. Persistent maternal hyperglycemia increases a woman's risk of having an infant with macrosomia and excessive maternal weight gain may also increase that risk.

Box 1
Criteria for testing for diabetes or prediabetes in asymptomatic adults, American Diabetes Association 2016

Overweight adults (BMI $\geq$25 kg/m^2 or $\geq$23 kg/m^2 in Asian Americans) with any of the following risk factors:

Physical inactivity; first-degree relative with diabetes; high-risk race/ethnicity including African American, Latino, Native American, Asian American, Pacific Islander; women who delivered a baby weighing >9 lb or were diagnosed with GDM; hypertension ($\geq$140/90 mm Hg or on therapy for hypertension); HDL cholesterol level $\leq$35 mg/dL and/or triglycerides >250 mg/dL; women with polycystic ovarian syndrome; hemoglobin A$_{1c}$ $\geq$5.7% or impaired fasting glucose on past testing; other clinical conditions associated with insulin resistance (eg, severe obesity, acanthosis nigricans); history of cardiovascular disease.

Abbreviations: BMI, body mass index; HDL, high-density lipoprotein.
Adapted from American Diabetes Association. Classification and diagnosis of diabetes. Sec. 2. In Standards of Medical Care in Diabetes – 2016. Diabetes Care 2016;39(Suppl 1):S16.

Box 2
Criteria for the diagnosis of type 2 diabetes, American Diabetes Association 2016

Fasting plasma glucose ≥126 mg/dL[a] or

2-h postglucose ≥200 mg/dL during a 75-g OGTT[a] or

Hemoglobin A_{1c} ≥6.5%[a] or

Classic symptoms of hyperglycemia with random plasma glucose ≥200 mg/dL[a]

[a] In the absence of unequivocal hyperglycemia, results should be confirmed by repeat testing.

Adapted from American Diabetes Association. Classification and diagnosis of diabetes. Sec. 2. In Standards of Medical Care in Diabetes – 2016. Diabetes Care 2016;39(Suppl 1):S14.

Macrosomia in turn is then associated with increased risk of operative delivery and with adverse neonatal outcomes including shoulder dystocia and its complications. Preeclampsia occurs more frequently in women with gestational diabetes. Polyhydramnios is more common among women with gestational diabetes. It does not seem to be associated directly with increased perinatal morbidity or mortality. The exact mechanism has never been determined, but a contributing factor is thought to be fetal polyuria. Although there are reports of stillbirths occurring among women with gestational diabetes, the mechanism is thought to be primarily related to poor glycemic control and does not seem to be increased compared with the general obstetric population and in women with good glycemic control.

The neonatal morbidities from mothers who have gestational diabetes include hypoglycemia, hyperbilirubinemia, hypocalcemia, hypomagnesia, polycythemia, respiratory distress, and cardiomyopathy. These risks are related to maternal hyperglycemia.

DIAGNOSIS OF GESTATIONAL DIABETES

In the United States a 50-g oral glucose challenge test (OGCT) and 100-g oral glucose tolerance test (OGTT) have been the standard to screen and diagnose GDM since O'Sullivan and coworkers[8] published a study in 1964 using these tests with collection of whole blood glucose measurements. Carpenter and Coustan[9] later converted O'Sullivan's whole blood glucose values to plasma glucose values with validation of the conversion by Sacks such that current guidelines use the Carpenter and Coustan plasma glucose values. However, the World Health Organization (WHO) had implemented a 75-g 2-hour OGTT for the diagnosis of GDM and an observational study by Sacks and colleagues[10] using those criteria showed a continuous relationship between fasting, 1-hour, and 2-hour OGTT values with birth-weight percentile and macrosomia. Later two randomized controlled trials using the WHO 75-g 2-hour OGTT showed that identifying and treating GDM reduced excess fetal growth and related complications.[11,12] In 2008 the HAPO (Hyperglycemia and Adverse Pregnancy Outcomes) trial, a multicenter, multinational epidemiologic study using the 75-g OGTT in nearly 25,000 pregnant women, showed at which level of mild hyperglycemia adverse pregnancy outcomes occurred. The study showed that increasing levels of plasma glucose are associated with birth weight greater than the 90th percentile; cord blood serum C peptide level greater than the 90th percentile; and to a lesser degree, primary cesarean deliveries and neonatal hypoglycemia.[13] Based on those results the International Association of

Diabetes and Pregnancy Study Groups (IADPSG) adopted the 75-g OGTT for the diagnosis of GDM. However, adoption of the 75-g OGTT with a lower threshold for the diagnosis of GDM was expected to increase the incidence of GDM from 5% to 6% to 15% to 20% because only one abnormal value is sufficient to make the diagnosis. The American College of Obstetricians and Gynecologists (ACOG) and later the National Institutes of Health Consensus Conference asserted that there were no adequately powered randomized controlled trials using the IADPSG/WHO criteria that showed improved pregnancy outcomes compared with the standard criteria. Additionally sited were the potentially negative consequences of identifying a large new group of women with GDM, including medicalization of pregnancy with increased interventions and cost, and the ease of screening with a 50-g OGCT such that the IADPSG/WHO criteria were not adopted by ACOG.

Therefore, the optimal screening/diagnostic approaches for gestational diabetes remain controversial. Universal screening is suggested because some women without risk factors develop GDM. The American Diabetes Association (ADA) and ACOG suggest that those at low risk for GDM need not be screened. Those at low risk include age less than 25 years; body mass index (BMI) 25 or less before pregnancy; not of Hispanic, African American, South or East Asian, or Pacific Islander decent; no first-degree relative with diabetes; no history of abnormal glucose tolerance; and no history of poor obstetric outcome.

Most US guidelines favor the two-step approach for screening, first administering a 50-g nonfasting OGCT test at 24 to 28 weeks, followed by a 100-g fasting OGTT for women who have a positive screening result.[14,15] However, clinicians may also use the IADPSG/WHO one-step approach with use of a 75-g 2-hour fasting OGTT with a lower threshold for diagnosis of gestational diabetes then with the two-step approach (**Table 1, Box 3**).[16]

The ADA recommends the use of either the one-step or two-step approach.[7,14–16] Based on the White Classification, women with GDM controlled by diet and exercise are labeled as GDM A1, whereas women with GDM who require insulin are labeled GDM A2.[9,16–19]

Table 1
Two-step approach for screening and diagnosis of gestational diabetes

Step 1: Perform a 50-g OGCT (nonfasting), with plasma glucose measurement at 1 h, at 24-to-28-wk gestation in women not previously diagnosed with overt diabetes.
If plasma glucose level 1 h after the load is ≥140 mg/dL proceed to a 100-g OGTT.

Step 2: The 100-g OGTT should be performed in a fasting state.
The diagnosis of GDM is made if two of the following four plasma glucose levels are met and either the Carpenter-Coustan or National Diabetes Data Group Criteria may be used:

	Carpenter-Coustan Criteria (mg/dL)	National Diabetes Data Group Criteria (mg/dL)
Fasting (h)	95	105
1	180	190
2	155	165
2	140	145

Adapted from Carpenter MW, Coustan DR. Criteria for screening tests for gestational diabetes. Am J Obstet Gynecol 1982;144(7):769; and Classification and diagnosis of diabetes mellitus and other categories of glucose intolerance. National Diabetes Data Group. Diabetes 1979;28(12):1039–57.

Box 3
One-step approach for screening and diagnosis of gestational diabetes

Perform a 75-g OGTT with plasma glucose measurement when patient is fasting and at 1 and 2 h, at 24-to-28-wk gestation in women not previously diagnosed with overt diabetes

The diagnosis of GDM is made when any one of the following plasma glucose values are met or exceeded:
   Fasting: 92 mg/dL
   1 h: 180 mg/dL
   2 h: 153 mg/dL

Adapted from Metzger BE, International Association of Diabetes and Pregnancy Study Groups Consensus Panel. International Association of Diabetes and Pregnancy Study Groups Recommendations on the Diagnosis and Classification of Hyperglycemia in Pregnancy. Diabetes Care 2010;33(3):676–82.

CLINICAL CARE
Lifestyle Management and Glucose Monitoring

Depending on the study population, 70% to 80% of women diagnosed with GDM by Carpenter-Coustan or National Diabetes Data Group criteria are controlled with lifestyle modification alone.[7]

Therefore, after the diagnosis of GDM, treatment should start with an education program to review medical nutrition therapy, glucose goals based on glucose monitoring, importance of physical activity, and weight management depending on pregestational weight. A suggested weight gain for overweight women is 15 to 25 pounds and for obese women 10 to 20 pounds.[7]

A diet with 33% to 40% carbohydrate with a preference for complex carbohydrate over simple carbohydrate with 20% protein, and 40% fat has been suggested to avoid excessive weight gain and reduce postprandial hyperglycemia.[20,21] Distributing calories between three meals and two to three snacks helps reduce postprandial glucose fluctuations.[14]

Glucose monitoring is recommended at four time points to include fasting and 1 or 2 hours after meals. Glucose targets from the Fifth International Workshop-Conference on Gestational Diabetes Mellitus[22] may be used:

- Fasting glucose ≤95 mg/dL and either
  - 1-hour postprandial ≤140 mg/dL or
  - 2-hour postprandial ≤120 mg/dL

For clarification, ACOG recommends a lower fasting goal of less than or equal to 90 mg/dL, and lower 1-hour postprandial glucose goal of less than or equal to 130 to 140 mg/dL, but same 2-hour postprandial less than or equal to 120 mg/dL for women with pregestational or type 2 diabetes.[14]

Regarding physical activity, it has been shown that adults with diabetes who are not pregnant and exercise have increased muscle mass and improved insulin sensitivity, but there are few published exercise trials in GDM with a large enough sample size to show a significant improvement in glucose levels. Despite that, a moderate exercise program is encouraged.[14]

Pharmacologic Therapy

When lifestyle intervention fails to maintain glucose levels at goal in GDM, the ADA considers insulin to be the first line treatment, whereas ACOG considers insulin and oral medications to be equivalent in efficacy with either being an appropriate choice for first-line therapy.[14,23]

Threshold values above which medication should be prescribed tend to be provider dependent. Possible thresholds used to start medications include more than two values after the same meal in a 2-week period above goal by 10 mg/dL or more, 50% of values in a given week are elevated above goal, fasting glucose greater than 90 mg/dL two or more occasions in a 2-week period, or 1-hour postprandial glucose values greater than 120 mg/dL.[12,24–26]

When needed, insulin provides the most rapid glucose control. Insulin may be started at a total daily dose of 0.7 to 1.0 units/kg actual body weight.[27] Obese women may require higher insulin dosing and insulin needs may double or triple during the pregnancy. If both the fasting and postprandial glucoses are above goal, half of the total daily dose may be given as the long-acting basal insulin and half may be given as rapid-acting insulin. The rapid acting insulin is split between the three meals and preferably dosed based on patients using an insulin/carbohydrate ratio (eg, one unit of rapid acting insulin per 15 g of carbohydrate). Basal insulins commonly used in pregnancy and typically dosed once a day include long-acting insulin analogues detemir and glargine, which are less likely to cause hypoglycemia than older basal insulins, such as neutral protamine Hagedorn (NPH), because of the relative lack of a peak.[28] Glargine has an increased affinity to the insulinlike growth factor-1 receptor, so there are theoretic concerns that it may contribute to adverse events in pregnancy, but adverse events have not been observed to date.[29–31] Because of the lack of adverse findings with glargine, women with pregestational diabetes may be continued on glargine during pregnancy, but it is suggested that those starting basal insulin in pregnancy start with NPH or detemir.[28,32]

NPH insulin is cheaper than the long-acting insulin analogues, but may predispose to hypoglycemia because of its peak levels by 6 to 7 hours of first dosing. Rapid-acting insulin analogues used in pregnancy include lispro and aspart and have replaced regular insulin at meals because of rapid onset and shorter duration of action, which provides better postprandial glucose control with less between-meal hypoglycemia.[28] A comparison of insulins is provided in **Table 2**. Dosing of insulin should be individualized and adjusted as needed. Patients benefit from frequent contact either by telephone, e-mail, or one-on-one visits with a certified diabetes educator.[28]

Two options of oral agents are available in the management of GDM and include metformin and glyburide. They have been shown to be effective with short-term safety in GDM with both being category B in pregnancy. Neither, however,

Table 2
Insulins used in diabetes and pregnancy

Type	Onset of action (h)	Peak of Action (h)	Duration of Action (h)
Insulin lispro	0.2–0.5	0.5–2	4–5
Insulin aspart	0.2–0.5	0.5–2	4–5
Regular insulin	0.5–1	2–3	6–8
NPH insulin	1.5–4	4–10	20
Insulin glargine	1–3	No peak	24
Insulin detemir	1–3	No peak	20

Adapted from Mooradian AD, Bernbaum M, Albert SG. Narrative review: a rational approach to starting insulin therapy. Ann Intern Med 2006;145:126; with permission.

has been approved by the US Food and Drug Administration for this indication. Evidence from randomized trials and observational studies of oral antidiabetic agents show that maternal glucose levels do not differ substantially between women treated with insulin and those treated with oral agents, and a meta-analysis showed no consistent evidence of an increase in adverse maternal outcomes with use of glyburide or metformin compared with insulin.[14] Because both oral agents cross the placenta and long-term safety data are not available, a role for counseling when prescribing these oral agents is suggested by the ADA and ACOG.[7,14]

Glyburide is a sulfonylurea that increases insulin secretion by binding to pancreatic β-cell adenosine triphosphate calcium channel receptors. It should not be used in patients with a sulfa allergy. The usual dose of glyburide is 2.5 to 20 mg per day in divided doses. From 20% to 40% of women on glyburide may require the addition of insulin to maintain glucose goals.[14] Metformin is a biguanide that reduces gluconeogenesis in the liver and stimulates glucose uptake in peripheral tissues. Because of its gastrointestinal side effect of diarrhea it is started at 500 mg once a day with food and may be titrated up to 2500 mg per day if tolerated (given as divided doses with meals). In the MiG trial,[33] half of the women randomized to metformin required insulin to achieve glucose goals and in a randomized controlled trial of glyburide versus metformin in GDM, 35% of the women randomized to metformin required insulin and 16% randomized to glyburide required insulin. This demonstrates that glyburide may be superior to metformin in GDM.[14]

Antenatal Fetal Testing

Women who have euglycemia with nutritional therapy and diet alone and who have no other maternal complications, such as macrosomia, preeclampsia, intrauterine growth restriction, or polyhydramnios, are not at increased risk of stillbirth.[34] Therefore performing antepartum testing and surveillance commencing at 32 weeks of gestation is not required. In those patients who require oral antihyperglycemic agents or insulin (GDM A2) to maintain euglycemia, initiation of antepartum testing at 32 weeks with twice-weekly testing is recommended. Some centers perform twice-weekly nonstress testing with amniotic fluid assessment twice weekly (modified biophysical profile). Other centers initiate antepartum testing surveillance weekly at 32 weeks and increase surveillance to twice weekly at 36 weeks gestation. ACOG has suggested antepartum fetal assessment for women with GDM and poor glycemic control without consensus about the management of those patients who are well controlled.

Assessment of Fetal Growth

Some clinicians perform an ultrasound evaluation shortly after the diagnosis of gestational diabetes is made and after an evaluation of maternal glycemic control. Many clinicians perform an ultrasound at the end of pregnancy for an estimated fetal weight and a discussion concerning options for timing and method of delivery. Unfortunately, no estimation of fetal growth performs well. All current methods indicate that there is a variance of approximately 20% in identifying the large for gestational age fetus.[35]

Timing of Delivery

One of the key issues related to the management of such patients is whether to induce labor and/or at what time. The potential benefits of induction are, in theory, the avoidance of late stillbirth and delivery-related complications from continued growth, especially if macrosomia has been identified. The disadvantages include the risk of induction with the possible need for cesarean section if the induction fails and for neonatal morbidity if the delivery is performed before 39 weeks. There are no data to support performing an induction of labor in a woman with well-controlled gestational diabetes with a suspicion of suspected fetal macrosomia or evolving macrosomia for concerns of a shoulder dystocia with its sequela. For those patients with GDM A1, current practice pattern is the beginning of a discussion about the possibility of induction when the patient reaches 40 0/7 weeks and then recommending induction by 41 weeks. The general consensus is those patients should not be induced before 39 weeks gestation. For those patients with GDM A2 taking either oral hypoglycemic agents or insulin, the recommendation is that those patients be delivered at 39 weeks gestation. The method of delivery should be based on a discussion relative to the risk of a shoulder dystocia based on a recently taken estimated fetal weight. A scheduled cesarean delivery to avoid birth trauma can be offered to these patients with an estimated fetal weight of more than 4500 g. This is the current recommendation of ACOG.[34] In patients without gestational diabetes, an elective cesarean delivery is reasonable when the estimated fetal weight is more than 5000 g.

In summary, there is no need for women with GDM A1 who are controlled by diet and lifestyle modification to be delivered early; an induction may be offered at 40 weeks gestation and induction recommended at 41 weeks. For those patients with type A2 diabetes requiring either oral hypoglycemic agents or insulin, the recommendation is that they be scheduled for an induction of labor at 39 weeks gestation and that a discussion concerning the potential risks of an induction of labor should occur. A single third-trimester ultrasound at or near the due date should be performed to evaluate for macrosomia and to then have a discussion of the risks and benefits of a cesarean delivery.

Intrapartum Glucose Management

Women with GDM A1 often require no intrapartum insulin. Those women with GDM A2 should be monitored every 1 to 2 hours during active labor and 5% dextrose or insulin infused as needed to maintain glucose control.[36] Consideration should be given to having women taking long-acting basal insulin reduce that dosing by half of their usual dose the night before and morning of delivery. Women with GDM rarely need oral agents or insulin after delivery, but before discharge short-term glucose monitoring is useful to ensure euglycemia.

Postpartum Care

At 6 to 12 weeks postpartum a 75-g 2-hour OGTT should be performed because up to 36% of women with GDM may have abnormal glucose tolerance.[14] Because GDM is associated with maternal risk for diabetes, women should be tested every 1 to 3 years thereafter if they passed the postpartum glucola, with the frequency of testing dependent on other risk factors, such as family history, prepregnancy BMI, and need for insulin or oral glucose-lowering agents during pregnancy. Ongoing screening may be achieved with any recommended screening test (hemoglobin A_{1c}, fasting plasma glucose, or 75-g OGTT using nonpregnant thresholds [ADA 2016]).[17] If women with past GDM are identified to have prediabetes (hemoglobin A_{1c} 5.7%–6.4%, impaired fasting glucose, or impaired glucose tolerance), both metformin and intensive lifestyle intervention prevent or delay progression to type 2 diabetes. In these women lifestyle intervention and metformin reduced progression to diabetes by 35% and 40%, respectively, over 10 years versus placebo.[37] Therefore, the ADA suggests that metformin be recommended for high-risk individuals (those with a history of GDM, BMI >35 kg/m^2, and/or progressive hyperglycemia) and/or rising hemoglobin A_{1c} despite lifestyle intervention.[38]

Contraception

The current 2016 Centers for Disease Control and Prevention recommendations[39] for contraception use for patients with a history of gestational diabetes is that none of the methods for contraception including oral contraceptives, both combined or progestin only, are contraindicated. Although any form of contraception is acceptable, the present recommendation is for the use of long acting reversible contraception (LARC) because of the minimal risk of unplanned pregnancy with that method of contraception. There is no evidence that using oral contraceptives either estrogen/progesterone or progesterone-only increases the risks of developing diabetes. These patients can breastfeed and should be encouraged to do so. The long-term benefits of performing breastfeeding on the development of type 2 diabetes have not yet been clarified.

SUMMARY

GDM and newly diagnosed type 2 diabetes in pregnancy are growing public health concerns related to the rise in obesity. To minimize complications to the mother and child, diagnosing and managing GDM is critical. However, the ideal screening, diagnostic testing, and management for GDM remains debated. Future randomized controlled trials need to address whether adopting stricter guidelines will improve pregnancy outcomes and what the optimal diet and treatments should be for women with GDM. Postpartum screening and long-term monitoring for diabetes is equally important given the increased risk for conversion to type 2 diabetes over time in those who have had GDM. Lifestyle intervention and metformin significantly reduce progression to type 2 diabetes in these women.

REFERENCES

1. Handwerger S, Freemark M. The roles of placental growth hormone and placental lactogen in the regulation of human fetal growth and development. J Pediatr Endocrinol Metab 2000;13:343.
2. Barbour LA. New concepts in insulin resistance of pregnancy and gestational diabetes: long-term implications for mother and offspring. J Obstet Gynaecol 2003;23:545.
3. Yamashita H, Shao J, Freidman J. Physiologic and molecular alterations in carbohydrate metabolism during pregnancy and gestational diabetes mellitus. Clin Obstet Gynecol 2000;43:87.
4. DeSisto CL, Kim SY, Sharma AJ. Prevalence estimates of gesational diabetes mellitus in the United States, Pregnancy Risk Assessment Monitoring System (PRAMS), 2007–2010. Prev Chronic Dis 2014;11:130–415.
5. Moyer VA. U.S. Preventive Services Task Force. Screening for gestational diabetes: U.S. Preventive Task Force recommendation statement. Ann Intern Med 2014;160:414.
6. Lawrence JM, Contreras R, Chen W, et al. Trends in the prevalence of preexisting diabetes and gestational diabetes mellitus among a racially/ethnically diverse population of pregnant women, 1999-2005. Diabetes Care 2008;31:899–904.

7. American Diabetes Association. Erratum. Classification and diagnosis of diabetes. Sec. 2. In Standards of Medical Care in Diabetes-2016. Diabetes Care 2016;39(Suppl. 1):S13–22.

8. O'Sullivan JB, Mahan CM, Charles D, et al. Screening criteria for high-risk gestational diabetic patients. Am J Obstet Gynecol 1973;116:895.

9. Carpenter MW, Coustan DR. Criteria for screening tests for gestational diabetes. Am J Obstet Gynecol 1982;144:768–73.

10. Sacks DA, Greenspoon JS, Abu-Fadil S, et al. Toward universal criteria for gestational diabetes: the 75-gram glucose tolerance test in pregnancy. Am J Obstet Gynecol 1995;172(2 Pt 1):607–14.

11. Crowther CA, Hiller JE, Moss JR, et al. Effect of treatment of gestational diabetes mellitus on pregnancy outcomes. N Engl J Med 2005;352:2477–86.

12. Landon MB, Spoing CY, Thom E, et al. A multicenter, randomized trial of treatment for mild gestational diabetes. N Engl J Med 2009;361(14):1339–48.

13. Metzger BE, Lowe LP, Dyer AR, et al, HAPO Study Cooperative Research Group. Hyperglycemia and adverse pregnancy outcomes. N Engl J Med 2008;358(19): 1991–2002.

14. Committee on Practice Bulletins-Obstetrics. Practice Bulletin N. 137: Gestational diabetes mellitus. Obstet Gynecol 2013;122(2 Pt 1):406–16.

15. National Institutes of Health consensus development conference statement: diagnosing gestational diabetes mellitus, March 4-6, 2013. Obstet Gynecol 2013; 122(2 Pt 1):358–69.

16. American Diabetes Association Standards of Medical Care in Diabetes-2016. Diabetes Care 2016;39(Suppl 1):S18–20.

17. White P. Pregnancy complicating diabetes. Am J Med 1949;7:609–16.

18. Metzger BE. International Association of Diabetes and Pregnancy Study Groups Consensus Panel. International Association of Diabetes and Pregnancy Study Groups recommendations on the diagnosis and classification of hyperglycemia in pregnancy. Diabetes Care 2010;33(3):676–82.

19. Classification and diagnosis of diabetes mellitus and other categories of glucose intolerance. National Diabetes Data Group. Diabetes 1979;28(12): 1039–57.

20. Mulford MI, Jovanovic-Peterson L, Peterson CM. Alternative therapies for the management of gestational diabetes. Clin Perinatol 1993;20:619–34.

21. Moses RG, Barker M, Winter M, et al. Can a low-glycemic index diet reduce the need for insulin in gestational diabetes mellitus? A randomized trial. Diabetes Care 2009;32:996–1000.

22. Metzger BE, Buchanan TA, Coustan DR. Summary and recommendations of the Fifth International Workshop-Conference on Gestational Diabetes Mellitus. Diabetes Care 2007;30(Suppl 2):S251–60.

23. American Diabetes Association Standards of Medical Care in Diabetes–2016. Diabetes Care 2016;39(suppl 1):S94–8.

24. Moore LE, Clokey D, Rappaport VJ, et al. Metformin compared with glyburide in gestational diabetes: a randomized controlled trial. Obstet Gynecol 2010;115(1): 55–9.

25. Hoffert Gilmartin AB, Ural S, Repke J. Gestational diabetes mellitus. Rev Obstet Gynecol 2008;1(3):129–34.

26. Garrison A. Screening, Diagnosis, and Management of Gestational Diabetes. Am Fam Physician 2015;91(7):460–7.

27. Kitzmiller J, Blockt J, Brown F, et al. Managing preexisting diabetes for pregnancy: summary of evidence and consensus recommendations for care. Diabetes Care 2008;31(5):1060–79.
28. Blumer I, Hadar E, Hadden D, et al. Diabetes and pregnancy: an Endocrine Society clinical practice guideline. J Clin Endocrinol Metab 2013;98(11): 4227–49.
29. Lambert K, Holt R. The use of insulin analogues in pregnancy. Diabetes Obes Metab 2013;15(10):888–900.
30. Lepercq J, Lin J, Hall GC. Meta-analysis of maternal and neonatal outcomes associated with the use of insulin glargine versus NPH insulin during pregnancy. Obstet Gynecol Int 2012;2012:649070.
31. Pollex E, Moreti ME, Loren G, et al. Safety of insulin glargine use in pregnancy: a systematic review and meta-analysis. Ann Pharmacother 2011; 45(1):9–16.
32. Mooradian AD, Bernbaum M, Albert SG. Narrative review: a rational approach to starting insulin therapy. Ann Intern Med 2006;145:125–34.
33. Rowan JA, Hague WM, Gao W, et al. Metformin versus insulin for the treatment of gestational diabetes. N Engl J Med 2008;358:2003–15.
34. Available at: http://www.acog.org/Resources-And-Publications/Practice-Bulletins/Committee-on-Practice-Bulletins-Obstetrics/Gestational-Diabetes-Mellitus.
35. Available at: http://www.acog.org/Resources-And-Publications/Practice-Bulletins/Committee-on-Practice-Bulletins-Obstetrics/Ultrasound-in-Pregnancy.
36. ACOG Committee Practice Bulletin. ACOG Practice Bulletin. Clinical Management Guidelines for Obstetrician-Gynecologists. Number 60, March 2005. Pregestational diabetes mellitus. Obstet Gynecol 2005;105(3):675–85.
37. Aroda VR, Christophi CA, Edelstein SL. The effect of lifestyle intervention and metformin on preventing or delaying diabetes among women with and without gestational diabetes: the Diabetes Prevention Program outcomes study 10-year follow-up. J Clin Endocrinol Metab 2015;100:1646–53.
38. American Diabetes Association Standards of Medical Care in Diabetes–2016. Diabetes Care 2016;39(suppl 1):S36–8.
39. Available at: https://www.cdc.gov/reproductivehealth/.../pdf/contraceptive_methods_508.pdf.

Updates on the Recognition, Prevention and Management of Hypertension in Pregnancy

CrossMark

Jessica R. Jackson, MD, MSBS[a], Anthony R. Gregg, MD, MBA[b],*

KEYWORDS

- Pregnancy • Hypertension • Criteria • Proteinuria • Aspirin • Treatment

KEY POINTS

- Proteinuria is sufficient but not necessary when defining preeclampsia, and the methods used to measure urinary protein levels have changed. Hypertension without proteinuria but with severe features is diagnostic.
- Low-dose aspirin is effective for the prevention of preeclampsia. The number needed to treat is 42 to 18 as risk changes from low to high.
- The recommended dose of low-dose acetylsalicylic acid for prevention of preeclampsia in the United States is 81 mg daily started at 12 to 28 weeks' gestation.
- Data suggest that treating mild to moderate blood pressure has maternal benefits; however, fetal/neonatal risk is uncertain.

INTRODUCTION

Practicing obstetrics care providers recognize that the management of patients with hypertension in pregnancy offers a myriad of rewards, challenges, and uncertainties. When addressing the uncertainties, clinicians resort to evidence-based guidance for answers. Types of evidence assume an established hierarchy with systematic reviews at the top[1] (**Fig. 1**). Systematic reviews often use meta-analysis to combine results from level II studies that report similar outcomes. Meta-analysis provides more certain point estimates and narrower confidence intervals. Clinically useful statistical point estimates derived from meta-analyses include number needed to treat (NNT). The

Disclosure: The authors have nothing to disclose.
[a] Maternal Fetal Medicine, Department of Obstetrics and Gynecology, University of Florida College of Medicine, PO Box 100294, Gainesville, FL 32610-0294, USA; [b] Maternal Fetal Medicine, Department of Obstetrics and Gynecology, University of Florida Health System, University of Florida College of Medicine, PO Box 100294, Gainesville, FL 32610-0294, USA
* Corresponding author.
E-mail address: greggar@ufl.edu

Obstet Gynecol Clin N Am 44 (2017) 219–230
http://dx.doi.org/10.1016/j.ogc.2017.02.007
0889-8545/17/© 2017 Elsevier Inc. All rights reserved.
obgyn.theclinics.com

Evidence Hierarchy

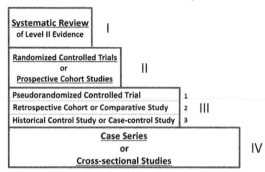

Fig. 1. Levels of evidence determine the weight given to studies that affect evidence-based clinical practice. Level I evidence is the highest level and takes advantage of randomized controlled trials and prospective cohort studies (level II evidence).

American College of Obstetricians and Gynecologists (ACOG) publication *Hypertension in Pregnancy* challenged previous criteria used to define preeclampsia, offered guidance on the use of low-dose acetylsalicylic acid (ASA) in pregnancy for the prevention of preeclampsia, and commented on the management of mild to moderate hypertension.[2] This article discusses these topics using the lens of already published meta-analyses.

DEFINING PREECLAMPSIA

In 1972, the ACOG established the classification scheme of hypertension-associated conditions in pregnancy (eg, gestational hypertension, preeclampsia, chronic hypertension, and chronic hypertension with superimposed preeclampsia).[2–4] Over the last 26 years, the defining features of preeclampsia were modified several times (**Table 1**). Recent modifications[2] emphasize proteinuria (300 mg/24 h) is sufficient but not necessary to make the diagnosis of preeclampsia. Furthermore, proteinuria can be established using a 24-hour urine collection or a urine protein/creatinine (P/C) ratio. Only when these methods are not available is a qualitative urine dipstick assay acceptable. The addition of the P/C ratio is sound, but the proposed threshold of 0.3 is open to critique. A systematic review, which included 7 studies and performed a receiver operator curve analysis, was used to derive clinically useful values for the P/C ratio[5] (**Table 2**). The investigators suggested that a value of less than 150 is useful as a screening tool to determine who should be tested using a 24-hour urine measurement, whereas a value greater than or equal to 600 could obviate the 24-hour specimen. Importantly, neither the 24-hour urine or P/C ratio are practical tests for immediate decision making and office practice. In these settings, a urine dipstick is appropriate.

The National Heart Lung and Blood Institute provided guidelines for the diagnosis of hypertension-associated conditions[6] and 10 years later revised the criteria.[7] Revisions included removal of edema as a criterion and specific blood pressure criteria were changed. Previously,[6] patients could be their own controls such that blood pressure comparisons before and after 20 weeks' gestation were used to establish patient-specific thresholds for disease (ie, 30 mm Hg increase in systolic or 15 mm Hg increase in diastolic after 20 weeks). The revision provided a single threshold value for all patients (140 mm Hg systolic or 90 mm Hg diastolic). It was determined that

Table 1
Features used to define preeclampsia between 1991 and 2013

	Hypertension	Proteinuria	Edema
NHLBI[6]	Criteria for significant increases in blood pressure established by comparing early pregnancy values with those measured after 20 wk	Dipstick: 1+ (30 mg/dL) Or 300 mg/24 h	Required
NHLBI[7]	Blood pressure: <140/90 mm Hg before 20 wk And Blood pressure: ≥140/90 mm Hg after 20 wk	Dipstick: 1+ (30 mg/dL) Or 300 mg/24 h	Not required
ACOG[2]	Blood pressure: <140/90 mm Hg before 20 wk And Blood pressure: ≥140/90 mm Hg after 20 wk	300 mg/24 h (a 24-h or timed specimen is recommended) Protein/creatinine: 0.3 (each measured mg/dL) Dipstick: discouraged unless last resort Or Not required[a]	Not required

Abbreviation: NHLBI, National Heart, Lung, and Blood Institute.
[a] When proteinuria is not identified (ie, not required), one of the defining criteria of severe disease (ie, platelet count <100,000/μL, serum transaminase levels twice upper limit of normal, serum creatinine level greater than or equal to 1.1 mg/dL or twice baseline with no renal disease, pulmonary edema, cerebral or visual disturbance) must be present.

blood pressure below this threshold was not likely to be associated with adverse pregnancy outcomes.[7] Blood pressure is a continuous trait variable and a danger in using absolute thresholds is that they are subject to being insensitive to patient-specific risk (eg, 140/90 mm Hg is greater than the 99% for some teenage girls).

PREVENTING PREECLAMPSIA

Disease prevention is a focus of health care delivery across nearly all disciplines of medicine. No change in activity, vitamin intake, or diet has an established benefit in preeclampsia prevention. After years of investigation, several meta-analyses

Table 2
Protein/creatinine ratio and results from receiver operator curve analysis

P/C Ratio (mg/g)[a]	Detection Rate[b] (%)	Sensitivity[b] (%)
130–150	90–99	33–65
300	81–98	52–99
600[c]–700	85–87	96–97

[a] Protein and creatinine levels are each measured in milligrams per deciliter according to ACOG. Therefore, values in this table are 3-fold higher because measurement of protein and creatinine was in milligrams per deciliter and grams per deciliter respectively.
[b] Detection rate and sensitivity are for a 24-hour specimen with 300 mg.
[c] 600 had a positive predictive value of 95%.
Data from Papanna R, Mann LK, Kouides RW, et al. Protein/creatinine ratio in preeclampsia: a systematic review. Obstet Gynecol 2008;112(1):135–44.

established the efficacy of low-dose aspirin for prevention of preeclampsia.[8–11] This article focuses on the meta-analysis published by the United States Preventive Services Task Force (USPTF),[9] which included only randomized controlled trials with a placebo and was restricted to those using 1 antiplatelet medication: aspirin. This analysis included women at increased risk of preeclampsia based on their medical and obstetric histories; furthermore, healthy nulliparous patients were excluded. The size of the studies varied and the baseline risk of preeclampsia ranged from 8% to 23%. **Box 1** shows the steps used to calculate the NNT and **Table 3** shows the NNT for each study included by the USPTF.

Based on available data, professional organizations suggested appropriate candidates for chemoprophylaxis with low-dose ASA (**Table 4**). Patients at the highest risk are those with a history of second-trimester preeclampsia and severe features (25%–65%).[12–17] The risk decreases when severe features are absent (5%–7%). Women with a prior normotensive pregnancy have the lowest risk (<1%) and healthy nulliparous women have a 2% to 4% risk. Assigning absolute risk to any given patient can be difficult, because of the many variables in play. Using a baseline risk of 10% to 23% and data from the USPTF study, the NNT ranged from 42 to 18.[9] **Table 5** shows data from 2 additional meta-analyses. The baseline risk before treatment has a profound impact on the NNT. Patients at higher risk for preeclampsia are more likely to derive a benefit from the use of low-dose ASA.

The studies included by the USPTF used dosages between 49 and 150 mg (see **Table 3**). There was no evidence of a dose-response relationship in the USPTF study.[9] However, a dosage of at least 75 mg/d had a greater benefit in reducing risk of preeclampsia than a dosage less than 75 mg/d (risk ratio [RR], 0.58 [95% confidence interval (CI), 0.36–0.95]; and RR, 0.85 [95% CI, 0.68–1.05] respectively), but confounding was considered possible. The dosing recommendations put forth by professional organizations and suggested by the USPTF are shown in **Table 4**. Although not specifically studied, the 81-mg dose was later recommended because of its availability in the United States and because it is within the aforementioned range (75–150 mg).[18] All studies in the USPTF analysis started low-dose ASA after 12 weeks' gestation. Timing of administration varied significantly across the studies considered (12–28 weeks), and there was no difference in the effect among patients starting treatment before or after 16 weeks' gestation.[9]

Box 1
The steps used to calculate the number needed to treat

Steps in determining NNT

1. Calculate the risk ratio (RR) using:
   a. Proportion of events among treated: events/exposed
   b. Proportion of events among controls (baseline risk): events/unexposed

2. Subtract 1 from the RR
   a. If number is positive, the event occurs more often
   b. If number is negative, the treatment is protective

3. Calculate the change in risk (absolute risk reduction [AR])
   a. If number is positive, the event occurs more often
   b. If number is negative, the treatment is protective

4. Calculate NNT
   AR = (RR − 1) baseline risk
   NNT = 1/AR; round up

Table 3
Data used in the United States Preventive Services Task Force meta-analysis to determine the number needed to treat

Study	N	ASA (mg)	Baseline Risk	EventsRx (%)	EventsCtrl (%)	RR[a]	Change in Risk[b]	New Risk[c]	NNT[d]
Grab et al,[26] 2000	48	100	0.10	3 out of 22 (14)	2 out of 21 (10)	1.40	0.04	0.14	25
Wallenburg et al,[27] 1986	44	60	0.30	0 out of 21 (0)	7 out of 23 (30)	0.00	−0.30	0.00	-
Caspi et al,[28] 1994	49	100	0.09	0 out of 24 (0)	2 out of 23 (9)	0.00	−0.09	0.00	-
Schiff et al,[29] 1989	65	100	0.23	1 out of 34 (3)	7 out of 31 (23)	0.13	−0.20	0.03	5
Vainio et al,[30] 2002	86	49	0.23	2 out of 43 (5)	10 out of 43 (23)	0.22	−0.18	0.05	6
Hermida et al,[31] 1997	100	100	0.14	3 out of 50 (6)	7 out of 50 (14)	0.43	−0.08	0.06	13
McParland et al,[32] 1990	100	75	0.19	1 out of 48 (2)	10 out of 52 (19)	0.11	−0.17	0.02	6
Villa et al,[33] 2013	121	100	0.18	8 out of 61 (13)	11 out of 60 (18)	0.72	−0.05	0.13	20
Viinikka et al,[34] 1993	197	50	0.11	9 out of 97 (1)	11 out of 100 (11)	0.09	−0.10	0.01	10
Ayala et al,[35] 2013	350	100	0.13	11 out of 176 (6)	22 out of 174 (13)	0.46	−0.07	0.06	14
Yu et al,[36] 2003	554	150	0.19	49 out of 276 (18)	52 out of 278 (19)	0.95	−0.01	0.18	100
Caritis et al,[37] 1998 MFMU	2505	60	0.20	226 out of 1254 (18)	250 out of 1249 (20)	0.90	−0.02	0.18	50
CLASP,[38] 1994	7974	60	0.08	267 out of 3992 (7)	302 out of 3982 (8)	0.88	−0.01	0.07	100
TOTAL	12,193								

Abbreviations: ASA, aspirin; EventsCtrl, events among those exposed to placebo; EventsRx, preeclampsia among those exposed to low-dose aspirin; N, study size; RR, risk ratio.

a RR is the proportion with preeclampsia in aspirin group/proportion with preeclampsia in placebo group.
b Change in risk = (RR − 1) baseline. Negative values indicate protective (eg, absolute risk reduction [AR] shown in **Box 1**).
c New risk was determined by adding/subtracting the baseline risk to the change in risk.
d NNT is determined by 1/change in risk. NNT values for risk that are increased are italicized. A dash (-) indicates that all exposed to aspirin experienced protection.

Data from Henderson JT, Whitlock EP, O'Connor E, et al. Low-dose aspirin for prevention of morbidity and mortality from preeclampsia: a systematic evidence review for the U.S. Preventive Services Task Force. Ann Intern Med 2014;160(10):695–703.

Table 4
Professional organization guidance on patients who are appropriate candidates for the use of low-dose aspirin to prevent preeclampsia

	USPTF[9]	ACOG[2]	NICE[25]	WHO[39]
	60–150 mg	60–80 mg	75 mg	75 mg
High (≥1)				
History of Preeclampsia	X	X	X	X
Multifetal Gestation[a]	X	X	—	X
Chronic Hypertension	X	X	X	X
Diabetes (Type 1 or Type 2)	X	X	X	X
Renal Disease	X	X	X	X
Autoimmune Disease	X	X	X	X
Moderate (>1)[b]				
Nulliparous	X	—	X	—
Age ≥40 y	—	—	X	—
>10 y IPI	X	—	X	—
First-degree Relative	X	—	X	—
BMI ≥35 kg/m^2	—	—	X	—
Multifetal Gestation[a]	—	—	X	—
Black Race	X	—	—	—
Low SES	X	—	—	—
Age >35 y	X	—	—	—
BMI >30 kg/m^2	X	—	—	—
Patient Born LBW	X	—	—	—
Prior APO	X	—	—	—

Abbreviations: APO, adverse pregnancy outcome (not specifically defined); BMI, body mass index; IPI, interpregnancy interval; LBW, low birth weight; NICE, National Institute for Health and Care Excellence (United Kingdom); SES, socioeconomic status (not specifically defined); WHO, World Health Organization.
   [a] Multifetal gestation is not a high-risk factor but is a moderate-risk factor in the NICE guidance.
   [b] Moderate-risk factors are those with less than 8% risk. NICE proposes 2 or more for aspirin prophylaxis.

TREATING HYPERTENSION

Across the United States, there is an emphasis on reducing the time from identification of severe-range blood pressure (≥160 mm Hg systolic or ≥110 mm Hg diastolic) to treatment in women with hypertension during pregnancy or the postpartum period. The goal is effective treatment within an hour.[19,20] Meta-analyses[21] show that treating mild to moderate hypertension during pregnancy reduces the risk of developing severe-range blood pressure (**Table 6**). The findings from these earlier studies were recently supported by data from an open-label, randomized controlled, multicenter trial. Patients with mild to moderate hypertension were managed with labetalol in order to achieve tight control versus less tight control.[22] There were no differences in composite neonatal or maternal outcomes. In this trial (N = 881) the proportion of women who developed preeclampsia was not different between the groups. This finding makes sense, because the development of proteinuria was not affected by tighter blood pressure treatment and defining features predated those put forth by ACOG in 2013 (see **Table 1**). However, severe hypertension was decreased in the tight-control group (adjusted odds ratio [OR], 1.80; 95% CI, 1.34–2.38) and fewer

Table 5
Relationship between baseline risk and number needed to treat from 3 published meta-analyses

Meta-analysis and Risk Stratification[a]	Baseline Risk	Pooled RR	Change in Risk[b]	Risk with Rx[c]	NNT
USPTF[9]					
Low	0.10	0.76	−0.02	0.08	42
Mid	0.18	0.76	−0.04	0.14	23
High	0.23	0.76	−0.06	0.17	18
Duley et al,[8] 2007					
Pooled	0.08	0.85	−0.01	0.07	83
Mod	0.06	0.85	−0.01	0.05	111
High	0.19	0.83	−0.03	0.16	31

Abbreviation: Rx, Medical Treatment.
[a] Risk stratification is unique to each study and derives from the studies included for analysis.
[b] Change in risk = (RR − 1)baseline (eg, AR shown in **Box 1**).
[c] Risk with treatment (new risk in **Table 3**) was determined by subtracting the change in risk from the baseline risk.

patients had low platelet counts (<100,000/μL; adjusted OR, 2.63; 95% CI, 1.15–6.05) or increased transaminase levels with symptoms (adjusted OR, 2.33; 95% CI, 1.05–5.16). Although not specifically evaluated in this study, it seems that application of recently proposed defining features might yield a reduction in preeclampsia when attempting to achieve tight blood pressure control for patients with mild to moderate hypertension. With a national emphasis on avoiding severe-range blood pressure to avert the risk of intracranial hemorrhage, it is logical to offer treatment to women with mild to moderate hypertension as long as there is no harm. In an early study of 2635 women, a reduction of 10 mm Hg in mean arterial pressure caused by blood pressure medication was associated with a 176-g decrease in birthweight.[23] In a meta-analysis[24] of β-blockers (eg, atenolol and labetalol) versus no treatment, there was an increased risk of small-for-gestational-age fetus (RR was 1.36; 95% CI, 1.02–1.82). In this analysis, 1 trial used atenolol as the preferred antihypertensive agent and 33% of patients exposed had a small-for-gestational-age fetus compared with no patients in the control group.

There are no convincing data to guide the blood pressure threshold for initiating treatment of mild to moderate hypertension. The UK National Institute for Health and Care Excellence (NICE) suggests 150 mm Hg systolic and/or 100 mm Hg diastolic.[25] Other professional organizations have not provided guidance. There are limited data indicating the optimal blood pressure target after initiation of medical intervention. In the published study described,[22] a target of 100 mm Hg diastolic was used for the group with less tight control and in the tight-control group a diastolic of 85 mm Hg was the target. There were no differences in infants born at the 10th or 3rd percentile (**Table 7**).

On balance, the maternal benefits of treating patients with mild to moderate hypertension seem to outweigh any neonatal risks. However, the paucity of data to guide the appropriate blood pressure threshold for the initiation of treatment or target values once treatment begins suggests a need for patient counseling. ACOG recommends not treating women with mild gestational hypertension or preeclampsia who have persistent blood pressure of less than 160 mm Hg systolic or 110 mm Hg diastolic; however, this guidance is subject to change in light of recently published data.

Table 6
Data from 2 meta-analyses showing that treatment of mild to moderate blood pressure protects against the development of severe-range blood pressure

Cochrane	N	Baseline Risk	Drug Exposure	EventsRx (%)	Events Ctrl (%)	RR[a]	Change in Risk[b]	New Risk[c]	NNT[d]
Severe HTN									
Magee et al,[24] 2003 (pooled)	1128	0.18	β-Blocker	36 out of 565 (6)	99 out of 563 (18)	0.36	−0.11	0.07	9
Abalos et al,[21] 2007 (pooled)	2558	0.20	β-Blocker, methyldopa, Ca++ channel blocker plus combinations of meds	129 out of 1336 (10)	242 out of 1222 (20)	0.49	−0.10	0.10	10

Abbreviations: EventsCtrl, events among those unexposed to treatment; EventsRx, severe-range blood pressure among those exposed to antihypertensive therapy.
[a] RR is the proportion with severe-range blood pressure in the treatment group/proportion with severe-range blood pressure in placebo group.
[b] Change in risk = (RR − 1)baseline (negative values indicate protective [eg, AR shown in **Box 1**]).
[c] New risk was determined by subtracting the baseline risk to the change in risk.
[d] NNT was determined by 1/change in risk.

Table 7
Data from a meta-analysis showing that treatment of mild to moderate blood pressure increases the risk of infants being small for gestational age

Cochrane	N	Drug Exposure	Baseline Risk	EventsRx (%)	EventsCtrl (%)	RR[a]	Change in Risk[b]	New Risk[c]	NNT[d]
Small for Gestational Age									
Magee et al,[24] 2003 (pooled)	1128	β-Blocker	0.10	99 out of 676 (15)	68 out of 670 (10)	1.39	0.04	0.07	25

Abbreviations: EventsRx, small for gestational age (<90%) among those exposed to antihypertensive therapy.
[a] RR is the proportion of small-for-gestational-age infants in the treatment group/proportion in placebo group.
[b] Change in risk = (RR − 1)baseline (negative values indicate protective [eg, AR shown in **Box 1**]).
[c] New risk was determined by subtracting the baseline risk to the change in risk.
[d] NNT was determined by 1/change in risk.

SUMMARY/DISCUSSION

Systematic reviews with meta-analysis represent the highest level of evidence used to guide clinical practice. The defining criteria used to diagnose preeclampsia have evolved, and are likely to continue to evolve. Proteinuria is sufficient but not necessary when defining preeclampsia. Hypertension without proteinuria but with severe features is diagnostic. The methods used to measure urinary protein level have changed. Proteinuria can now be determined using the urine P/C ratio, whereas qualitative urine dipstick assessment has become less favored. The gold standard remains the 24-hour urine test. The efficacy of low-dose aspirin in preventing preeclampsia is a function of baseline risk, with the NNT suggesting 42 to 18 as risk changes from low to high. For practical reasons, the recommended dosage in the United States is 81 mg daily starting at 12 to 28 weeks' gestation. Data suggest that treating mild to moderate blood pressure has clear maternal benefits with very little fetal or neonatal risk. The appropriate blood pressure to trigger the initiation of therapy and the target blood pressure once treatment begins are unknown.

ACKNOWLEDGMENTS

The authors thank Marsha Harben for her assistance with this article.

REFERENCES

1. Australian Government National Health and Medical Research Council. NHMRC additional levels of evidence and grades for recommendations for developers of guidelines. 2009. Available at: https://www.nhmrc.gov.au/_files_nhmrc/file/guidelines/developers/nhmrc_levels_grades_evidence_120423.pdf. Accessed December 15, 2016.
2. American College of Obstetricians and Gynecologists. Task Force on Hypertension in Pregnancy. ACOG Hypertension in Pregnancy Task Force. Washington, DC: American College of Obstetricians and Gynecologists; 2013.
3. Vanek M, Sheiner E, Levy A, et al. Chronic hypertension and the risk for adverse pregnancy outcome after superimposed pre-eclampsia. Int J Gynecol Obstet 2004;86:7–11.
4. Hughes EC. Obstetric terminology. In: Mitchell Perry H Jr, editor. Lifelong management of hypertension. Philadelphia: Springer Science and Business Media; 1972. 442–423.
5. Papanna R, Mann LK, Kouides RW, et al. Protein/creatinine ratio in preeclampsia: a systematic review. Obstet Gynecol 2008;112:135–44.
6. National High Blood Pressure Education Program Working Group report on high blood pressure in pregnancy. Am J Obstet Gynecol 1990;163(5 Pt 1):1691–712.
7. National Heart Lung and Blood Institute. Working Group report on high blood pressure in pregnancy. Bethesda (MD): National Institutes of Health; 2000.
8. Duley L, Henderson-Smart DJ, Meher S, et al. Antiplatelet agents for preventing pre-eclampsia and its complications (review). Cochrane Database Syst Rev 2007;(2):CD004659.
9. Henderson JT, Whitlock EP, O'Connor E, et al. Low-dose aspirin for prevention of morbidity and mortality from preeclampsia: a systematic evidence review for the U.S. Preventive Services Task Force. Ann Intern Med 2014;160:695–703.
10. Askie LM, Duley L, Henderson-Smart DJ, et al. Antiplatelet agents for prevention of pre-eclampsia: a meta-analysis of individual patient data. Lancet 2007;369: 1791–8.

11. Bujold E, Roberge S, Lacasse Y, et al. Prevention of preeclampsia and intrauterine growth restriction with aspirin started in early pregnancy. Obstet Gynecol 2010;116:402–14.

12. Sibai BM, El-Nazer A, Gonzalez-Ruiz A. Severe preeclampsia-eclampsia in young primigravid women: subsequent pregnancy outcome and remote prognosis. Am J Obstet Gynecol 1986;155:1011–6.

13. van Rijn BB, Hoeks LB, Bots ML, et al. Outcomes of subsequent pregnancy after first pregnancy with early-onset preeclampsia. Am J Obstet Gynecol 2006;195: 723–8.

14. Sibai BM, Sarinoglu MB. Severe preeclampsia in the second trimester: recurrence risk and long-term prognosis. Am J Obstet Gynecol 1991;165:1408–12.

15. Gaugler-Senden IPM, Berends AL, de Groot CJM, et al. Severe, very early onset preeclampsia: subsequent pregnancies and future parental cardiovascular health. Eur J Obstet Gynecol Reprod Biol 2008;140:171–7.

16. Campbell DM, Macgillivray I, Carr-Hill R. Pre-eclampsia in second pregnancy. Br J Obstet Gynaecol 1985;92:131–40.

17. Xiong X, Fraser WD, Demianczuk NN. History of abortion, preterm, term birth, and risk of preeclampsia: a population-based study. Am J Obstet Gynecol 2002;187:1013–8.

18. LeFevre ML. Low-dose aspirin use for the prevention of morbidity and mortality from preeclampsia: U.S. Preventive Services task force recommendation statement. Ann Intern Med 2014;161:819–26.

19. Florida Perinatal Quality Collaborative. 2016. Available at: http://health.usf.edu/publichealth/chiles/fpqc/hip. Accessed December 15, 2016.

20. California Maternal Quality Care Collaborative. 2016. Available at: https://www.cmqcc.org/resources-tool-kits/toolkits/preeclampsia-toolkit. Accessed December 15, 2016.

21. Abalos E, Duley L, Steyn DW, et al. Antihypertensive drug therapy for mild to moderate hypertension during pregnancy. Cochrane Database Syst Rev 2007;(1):CD002252.

22. Magee LA, von Dadelszen P, Rey E, et al. Less-tight versus tight control of hypertension in pregnancy. N Engl J Med 2015;372:407–17.

23. von Dadelszen P, Magee LA. Fall in mean arterial pressure and fetal growth restriction in pregnancy hypertension: an updated metaregression analysis. J Obstet Gynaecol Can 2002;24:941–5.

24. Magee LA, Cham C, Waterman AO, et al. Hydralazine for treatment of severe hypertension in pregnancy: meta-analysis. BMJ 2003;327:1–10.

25. NICE National Institute for Health and Care Excellence. Hypertension in pregnancy: diagnosis and management. NICE-National institute for Health and Care Excellence Guideline. 2010. Available at: http://nice.org.uk/guidance/cg107.

26. Grab D, Paulus WE, Erdmann M, et al. Effects of low-dose aspirin on uterine and fetal blood flow during pregnancy: results of a randomized, placebo-controlled, double-blind trial. Ultrasound Obstet Gynecol 2000;15:19–27.

27. Wallenburg HC, Dekker GA, Makovitz JW, et al. Low-dose aspirin prevents pregnancy-induced hypertension and pre-eclampsia in angiotensin-sensitive primigravidae. Lancet 1986;327:1–3.

28. Caspi E, Raziel A, Sherman D, et al. Prevention of pregnancy-induced hypertension in twins by early administration of low-dose aspirin: a preliminary report. Am J Reprod Immunol 1994;31:19–24.

29. Schiff E, Peleg E, Goldenberg M, et al. The use of aspirin to prevent pregnancy-induced hypertension and lower the ratio of thromboxane A2 to prostacyclin in relatively high risk pregnancies. N Engl J Med 1989;321:351–6.

30. Vainio M, Kujansuu E, Iso-Mustajarvi M, et al. Low dose acetylsalicylic acid in prevention of pregnancy-induced hypertension and intrauterine growth retardation in women with bilateral uterine artery notches. BJOG 2002;109:161–7.

31. Hermida RC, Ayala DE, Iglesias M, et al. Time-dependent effects of low-dose aspirin administration on blood pressure in pregnant women. Hypertension 1997;30:589–95.

32. McParland P, Pearce JM, Chamberlain GV. Doppler ultrasound and aspirin in recognition and prevention of pregnancy-induced hypertension. Lancet 1990; 335:1552–5.

33. Villa PM, Kajantie E, Raikkonen K, et al. Aspirin in the prevention of pre-eclampsia in high-risk women: a randomised placebo-controlled PREDO trial and a meta-analysis of randomised trials. BJOG 2013;120:64–74.

34. Viinikka L, Hartikainen-Sorri AL, Lumme R, et al. Low dose aspirin in hypertensive pregnant women: effect on pregnancy outcome and prostacyclin-thromboxane balance in mother and newborn. Br J Obstet Gynaecol 1993;100:809–15.

35. Ayala DE, Ucieda R, Hermida RC. Chronotherapy with low-dose aspirin for prevention of complications in pregnancy. Chronobiol Int 2013;30:260–79.

36. Yu CK, Papageorghiou AT, Parra M, et al. Randomized controlled trial using low-dose aspirin in the prevention of pre-eclampsia in women with abnormal uterine artery Doppler at 23 weeks' gestation. Ultrasound Obstet Gynecol 2003;22: 233–9.

37. Caritis S, Sibai B, Hauth J, et al. Low-dose aspirin to prevent preeclampsia in women at high risk. National Institute of Child Health and Human Development Network of Maternal-Fetal Medicine Units. N Engl J Med 1998;338:701–5.

38. CLASP: a randomised trial of low-dose aspirin for the prevention and treatment of pre-eclampsia among 9364 pregnant women. CLASP (Collaborative Low-dose Aspirin Study in Pregnancy) Collaborative Group. Lancet 1994;343(8898): 619–29.

39. WHO recommendations for prevention and treatment of pre-eclampsia and eclampsia. 2011. Available at: http://apps.who.int/iris/bitstream/10665/44703/1/ 9789241548335_eng.pdf. Accessed December 15, 2016.

Obstetric Emergencies

Shoulder Dystocia and Postpartum Hemorrhage

Joshua D. Dahlke, MD[a],*, Asha Bhalwal, MD[b],
Suneet P. Chauhan, MD[b]

KEYWORDS

- Obstetric emergencies • Postpartum hemorrhage • Shoulder dystocia • Risk factors
- Management

KEY POINTS

- Although certain risks for shoulder dystocia and postpartum hemorrhage exist, many cases occur in the absence of these factors.
- Early identification, communication, and familiarity with management options for both conditions can significantly minimize the morbidity associated with these complications.
- Institutional protocols and algorithms have been developed to familiarize caregivers with prevention and management options for these conditions.

INTRODUCTION

Shoulder dystocia and postpartum hemorrhage represent two of the most common emergencies faced in obstetric clinical practice, both requiring prompt recognition and management in order to avoid significant morbidity or mortality. Although certain risks for shoulder dystocia and postpartum hemorrhage exist, many cases occur in the absence of these factors. Early identification, communication, and familiarity with management options for both conditions can significantly minimize the morbidity associated with these complications.

Institutional protocols and algorithms for the prevention and management of both shoulder dystocia and postpartum hemorrhage have become mainstays for clinicians. The goal of this review is to summarize the diagnosis, incidence, risk factors, and management of shoulder dystocia and postpartum hemorrhage.

Disclosure Statement: The authors have nothing to disclose.

[a] Division of Maternal-Fetal Medicine, Department of Obstetrics and Gynecology, Nebraska Methodist Women's Hospital and Perinatal Center, 717 North 190th Plaza, Suite 2400, Omaha, NE 68022, USA; [b] Division of Maternal-Fetal Medicine, Department of Obstetrics, Gynecology, and Reproductive Sciences, UT Health-University of Texas Medical School at Houston, Houston, TX, USA
* Corresponding author.
E-mail address: joshuadahlke@gmail.com

SHOULDER DYSTOCIA
Definition

According to the American College of Obstetricians and Gynecologists (ACOG), shoulder dystocia is defined as the inability for the clinicians to complete the delivery of the fetus with gentle downward traction after the emergence of the head. Although the definition is subjective in nature, relief of an impacted shoulder against symphysis pubis requires additional ancillary maneuvers to deliver the fetus.[1]

The objective definition of shoulder dystocia is a prolongation of head-to-body time interval of more than 60 seconds.[2] Despite the numerical nature of this definition in the literature, it is not acknowledge by the ACOG or by the Royal College of Obstetricians and Gynecologists (RCOG).[1,3,4]

Incidence

In a review article on the definition and incidence of shoulder dystocia among 28 publications with more than 16 million total births, the rate of shoulder dystocia was 0.4%.[5] Since 2000, among all births, the rate of shoulder dystocia approximates 1.4% if publications reliant on *International Classification of Diseases* (*ICD*) codes are excluded. During vaginal delivery, the reported likelihood of shoulder dystocia in 15 publications was 0.7% overall, though it was higher among reports from the United States (1.4%) than other countries (0.6%).[5]

Four studies stratified the rate of shoulder dystocia among diabetic patients (gestational or pregestational) and nondiabetic patients. Notably, the rate of shoulder dystocia was 1.9% for women with diabetes compared with 0.6% for those without, a relative difference of 216%. Despite this increased risk, the 4 publications note that only 4% of the reported shoulder dystocias occurred in those with gestational or pregestational diabetes.[5]

Further, 6 of the studies reviewed provided the rate of shoulder dystocia among women with and without operative (vacuum or forceps) vaginal deliveries. The rate of shoulder dystocia was 2.0% for those who had operative birth and 0.6% if they did not, a relative difference of 254%. In these 6 reports, 21% of the shoulder dystocias occurred following operative vaginal birth.

Risk Factors

In addition to the aforementioned gestational or pregestational diabetes and operative vaginal delivery, obtaining a history of prior shoulder dystocia may be the most important risk factor. Simply put, shoulder dystocia reoccurs. A history of prior shoulder dystocia, which is knowable at first prenatal visit, may have one of the highest likelihood of future occurrence of an impacted shoulder. Of 9 studies that provided the rate of shoulder dystocia, recurrence was noted in 12% of vaginal births. Not only is recurrent shoulder dystocia more common but it also seems to be more morbid for the neonate. Although the rate of neonatal brachial plexus palsy is 19 of 1000 in those with the first shoulder dystocia, it increases to an estimated 45 of 1000 with recurrent shoulder dystocia, a relative increase of 136%.[6] An important caveat to these estimates, however, is the fact that true incidence of recurrent shoulder dystocia remains unknown because of many clinicians and patients not attempting a trial of labor and delivering via cesarean in subsequent pregnancies when a complicated delivery or neonatal injury occurs.[1]

The ACOG's practice bulletin on shoulder dystocia recognizes 10 risk factors that can be categorized into antepartum or intrapartum[1] (**Table 1**). Antepartum risks include a history of prior shoulder dystocia, history of macrosomia (birth weight of

Table 1
Summary of shoulder dystocia diagnosis, incidence, risk factors, and management

	Comments	References
Diagnosis	• Vaginal delivery that is not effectuated with gentle downward traction and requires additional ancillary maneuvers • Head-to-body time interval of more than 60 s	American College of Obstetricians and Gynecologists,[1] 2002 Spong et al,[2] 1995
Incidence	• Among all births: 0.4% • With vaginal deliveries: 1.4% • Among diabetic patients: 1.9% • With operative vaginal deliveries: 2.0%	Hansen & Chauhan,[5] 2014
Risk factors	• Antepartum ○ History of prior shoulder dystocia ○ History of macrosomia: birth weight of 4000 g (8 lb 13 oz or more) ○ Obesity ○ Multiparity ○ Diabetes: pregestational or gestational ○ Gestational age ≥41 wk • Intrapartum ○ Labor induction ○ Epidural anesthesia ○ Operative vaginal delivery ○ Macrosomia	American College of Obstetricians and Gynecologists,[1] 2002
Treatment (management)	• Initial or simple maneuvers ○ Summon additional assistance ○ McRoberts maneuver ○ Suprapubic pressure • Internal maneuvers or maternal position change ○ All-fours position if feasible ○ Extraction of the posterior arm ○ Rotation of the posterior shoulder ○ Rotation of the anterior shoulder • Third-line maneuvers ○ Zavanelli ○ Cleidotomy: fracture of the clavicle ○ Symphysiotomy	American College of Obstetricians and Gynecologists,[1] 2002; Royal College of Obstetricians and Gynecologists,[3] 2012; Hansen & Chauhan,[5] 2014; Bruner et al,[14] 1998

4000 g [8 lb 13 oz or more]), maternal obesity, multiparity, pregestational or gestational diabetes, and gestational age of 41 weeks or greater. Intrapartum risks include labor induction, epidural anesthesia, and operative vaginal delivery.

Despite these multiple known risk factors, it is noteworthy that most shoulder dystocias are uncommon, unpredictable, and unpreventable. Gross and colleagues[7] reported a mathematical model suggesting that only 16% of all shoulder dystocias with concomitant neonatal trauma could be predicted. When considering 17 antepartum and intrapartum variables, this model attests to the unlikelihood for clinicians to identify the woman who will have shoulder dystocia and, most importantly, predict neonatal morbidity, such as neonatal brachial plexus palsy. In summary, although risk factors for shoulder dystocia are elucidated, they are insufficiently sensitive to be clinically useful to avert neonatal injury, like persistent neonatal brachial plexus palsy.

Prevention

As previously mentioned, the risk of reoccurrence in women with previous shoulder dystocia may be as high as 12% and the second shoulder dystocia is more likely to be associated with injury to the newborn than the first shoulder dystocia.[1,4,6] Most subsequent deliveries, however, do not result in shoulder dystocia, thus, leaving clinicians and patients with a difficult decision. To prevent injury with subsequent deliveries, cesarean delivery should be discussed as an option; but, as noted in the ACOG's practice bulletin, its benefit is uncertain.[1] Clinicians should consider the status of diabetes, estimated fetal weight, progression of labor, and if possible avoid operative vaginal deliveries. The recognized risks associated with primary cesarean delivery should also be considered and discussed, with the ultimate delivery route appropriate after proper counseling.

To avert shoulder dystocia, clinicians may undertake unnecessary primary cesarean for suspected macrosomia. Up to 4% of primary cesarean delivery are done for suspected macrosomia.[8] Vagaries exist with regard to sonographically estimating fetal weight.[9] Furthermore, the risk of maternal death with cesarean delivery and the risk of persistent neonatal brachial plexus palsy with vaginal births are similar, making the excessive rate of cesarean delivery for estimated fetal weight unwarranted in most case.[8,10] Therefore, the ACOG, RCOG, and the Society of Maternal-Fetal Medicine (SMFM) recommend that cesarean delivery for the indication of presumed macrosomia should be offered only to those with a sonographic estimated fetal weight greater than 5000 g in nondiabetic patients and 4500 g in diabetic patients.[1,3,8]

Management

Both the ACOG and RCOG have national guidelines on shoulder dystocia, and they have slightly different suggestions on how to resolve the impacted shoulder.[1,3] When faced with a shoulder dystocia, it is incumbent on the clinician to remain calm and communicate clearly the situation. The first step, according to the RCOG, is to call for additional help. The support team may include additional nurses, midwives, obstetricians, maternal-fetal medicine subspecialist, neonatal resuscitation team, and anesthetist. When additional assistants arrive, they should be clearly informed that this is a situation of shoulder dystocia. According to Grobman and colleagues,[11] the emergency call for help represents an important component of a shoulder dystocia protocol associated with a significant decrease in the likelihood of neonatal brachial plexus palsy.

According to the ACOG, the performance of the McRoberts maneuver should be the initial step to resolve shoulder dystocia. This maneuver consists of hyperflexion and abduction of the hips, which putatively leads to cephalad rotation of the symphysis pubis and flattening of the lumbar lordosis, thus, mechanistically relieving the impacted shoulder.[1] In contemporary practice in the United States, women who deliver vaginally are often already in the McRoberts position rather than lithotomy despite no evidence that this preventive positioning decreases the rate of shoulder dystocia in all deliveries.[3] Thus, when a true shoulder dystocia does occur, it may be reasonable to ensure that the woman is in McRoberts position and if a family member is assisting with the maternal position, replaced by a member of the labor and delivery staff.

In addition to or in conjunction with the McRoberts maneuver, suprapubic pressure may be used to assist with the delivery of the impacted shoulder. The RCOG's guideline remarks that suprapubic pressure improves the effectiveness of McRoberts.[3] The mechanism of application of pressure over the symphysis presumably decreases the fetal bisacromial diameter and rotates the anterior fetal shoulder into the wider oblique pelvic diameter. The shoulder is then freed to slip underneath the symphysis pubis with the aid of routine axial traction.[3] Once these two simple maneuvers have been applied, routine or gentle traction in the axial direction may be applied to assess if the anterior shoulder has been released.[3] In 2 large multicenter studies, the use of McRoberts with or without suprapubic pressure relieved about two-thirds of the shoulder dystocia.[12,13]

If these initial maneuvers are unsuccessful in relieving the shoulder dystocia, clinicians have a choice of repositioning laboring patients to their hands and knees (all-fours maneuver) or performed internal manipulation of the fetus. The all-fours maneuver in one case series was demonstrated as a rapid, safe, and effective technique that resolved 83% of shoulder dystocia cases without any further maneuvers.[14] Although the RCOG's guideline considers this technique useful for mobile women after the simple maneuvers were unsuccessful, the ACOG's practice bulletin does not even mention it, perhaps because of the rarity of its use in the United States.[1,3] In a secondary analysis of the Consortium on Safe Labor, Hoffman and colleagues[12] noted that among 2000 shoulder dystocias, the all-fours maneuver was used in 22 instances or about 1% of cases of impacted shoulders. Regardless of infrequent utilization in the United States, it is notable that the all-fours technique reportedly has a success rate of more than 80% and could be considered if feasible and if the clinicians, including the nurses, are experienced.[14]

In the aforementioned secondary analysis, Hoffman and colleagues[12] found that delivery of the posterior shoulder was associated with an 84% rate of achieving delivery compared with 24% to 72% with other internal maneuvers. The rate of neonatal injury was similar whether the posterior arm was extracted (8%) or other maneuvers were used (6%–14%). Thus, they recommend extraction of the posterior arm if McRoberts and suprapubic pressure are unsuccessful.[12] Mechanistically, delivery of the posterior arm reduces the diameter of the fetal shoulder to accomplish delivery, which can be accomplished by grasping the fetal wrist and gently withdrawing the posterior arm in a straight line. This maneuver is associated with fracture of the neonatal humerus; however, this may be secondary to the refractory nature of shoulder dystocia rather than the maneuver itself.[3]

If the shoulder dystocia persists or if extraction of the posterior is not feasible, manual rotation of the neonatal shoulder should be attempted. Previous eponyms attributed to those credited to these maneuvers, Woods screw (anterior shoulder abduction) and Rubin maneuvers (posterior shoulder rotation), should be avoided.[3] In contrast and because the most spacious aspect of the pelvis is the sacral hallow, vaginal access should be initially attempted posteriorly. To accomplish this, the woman should be at the end of the bed, which allows the clinician's entire hand to enter posteriorly. Pressure applied to the posterior aspect of the posterior shoulder abducts the shoulder, and rotation of the shoulder in oblique diameter assists in resolving the impaction. If neither the extraction of the posterior arm nor the rotation of the posterior shoulder effectuates delivery, applying similar pressure to the posterior aspect of the anterior and rotation in a similar oblique diameter may be attempted.[3]

After the initial and internal maneuvers are performed and a shoulder dystocia persists, most clinicians are in an exceedingly unusual situation, as these resolve more than 99% of all should dystocias. Preferably the assistance that was summoned at the initial diagnosis of shoulder dystocia has arrived and can assist with effectuating the delivery. Neither the ACOG's nor the RCOG's guidelines on the topic comment on whether the maneuvers should be reattempted by another clinician. Considering the complexity of third-line maneuvers and the clinical situation, it may be reasonable to retry the initial maneuvers with the summoned assistance.

Third-line maneuvers to resolve shoulder dystocia include cleidotomy (intentional clavicular fracture), symphysiotomy (separation of the cartilage of the pubic symphysis), and the Zavanelli maneuver (cephalic replacement and subsequent cesarean delivery). The most commonly described of these remains the Zavanelli maneuver, although it is used quite rarely as exemplified by combining the results of 2 multicenter studies. Combined data of Hoffman and colleagues[12] and Chauhan and colleagues[13] indicate that among 178,735 deliveries, with 3195 (2%) shoulder dystocias, the Zavanelli maneuver was used once or 0.001% of all deliveries. Lastly, it is worth noting that maternal safety with the Zavanelli maneuver is unknown, and the procedure is associated with neonatal hypoxic ischemic injury and brachial plexus palsy.

In summary, shoulder dystocia remains an uncommon, unpredictable, and unpreventable obstetric situation, which can be managed with appropriate maneuvers. Institutional protocols have shown improved neonatal outcomes. Communication remains paramount when faced with this obstetric emergency. Preparation and understanding of initial, internal, and rarely used third-line maneuvers will allow the clinician to approach shoulder dystocia in a calm and stepwise manner. With experience, shoulder dystocia can be approached with resolve and confidence and not as a nightmare for clinicians.[15,16]

POSTPARTUM HEMORRHAGE
Diagnosis

Significant variation exists regarding the amount of blood loss that constitutes clinically relevant postpartum hemorrhage. Therefore, a previous review of national guidelines on the topic demonstrated a variety of acceptable definitions for postpartum hemorrhage.[17] Compounding this problem further is the fact that the most common method for estimating blood loss, the delivering provider visually estimating the amount of blood loss, has been shown to be highly inaccurate by underestimating blood loss by up to 30% to 50%.[18]

One definition endorsed by multiple national organizations, including the ACOG, SMFM, the American College of Nurse-Midwives (ACNM), the Association of Women's Health, Obstetric and Neonatal Nurses (AWHONN), and the California Maternal Quality Care Collaborative (CMQCC), is the following: a cumulative blood loss of greater than 1000 mL or blood loss accompanied by sign/symptoms of hypovolemia within 24 hours following the birth process.[19,20] An alternative definition used by the World Health Organization (WHO) is blood loss of 500 mL or more within 24 hours after birth.[21] One possible explanation for the variation between these definitions may be the difference in resource-rich versus resource-poor populations of the organizations' respective intended audiences. For purposes of this review, discussion of postpartum hemorrhage in the setting of a resource-rich environment is reviewed.

Because of the inaccuracy of visual estimates of blood loss, one effort to improve quality and postpartum hemorrhage recognition involves support staff to formally measure and quantify cumulative blood loss after every birth. Although requiring more resources than qualitative measurement, the goal is to more accurately assess actual blood loss and minimize delay in resuscitative measures when necessary. This method for blood loss measurement is supported and extensively reviewed by the AWHONN and the preferred measurement method in the CMQCC's obstetric hemorrhage toolkit.[20,22]

Incidence

Postpartum hemorrhage occurs in an estimated 4% to 6% of all pregnancies.[23,24] The RCOG estimates 3 of 1000 experience severe hemorrhage, defined as receipt of blood transfusion, hysterectomy, and/or surgical repair of the uterus.[25] Of those who experience postpartum hemorrhage, by far the most common cause is uterine atony, or the inability of the uterus to contract effectively, which accounts for more than 80% of cases. Other common culprits include retained placenta tissue, vaginal or cervical trauma, and known or developing coagulopathy.[23]

Risk Factors

Many risk factors exist that may increase a woman's chance of postpartum hemorrhage. These risks include preexisting conditions that may be known or apparent in the antepartum period, placental factors, or those that become apparent in the course of labor. It is important for the clinician to realize, however, that like shoulder dystocia, most women who experience postpartum hemorrhage do not have any known risk factors.

Preexisting factors identified by the ACOG and RCOG's national guidelines include history of postpartum hemorrhage, preeclampsia, overdistended uterus (macrosomia, twins, hydramnios), obesity, anemia, and Asian or Hispanic ethnicity. Antepartum conditions include prolonged, augmented, or rapid labor; episiotomy; operative delivery; infection; and induction of labor. Finally, placental factors include placenta abruption, previa, retained placenta, and abnormal placentation.[17,23,25] Of the risk factors reviewed earlier, the RCOG's guideline on postpartum hemorrhage specifies those conditions that put a woman at highest risk and includes suspected or proven placental abruption (odds ratio [OR] 13; 99% confidence interval [CI], 7.6–12.9), known placenta previa (OR 12; 99% CI, 7.2–23), multiple pregnancy (OR 5; 99% CI, 3.0–6.6), and preeclampsia (OR 4; 99% CI, not specified).[25]

Prevention

Preemptive measures to minimize postpartum hemorrhage have been one of the most studied subjects in obstetrics literature. Much of this inquiry has focused on the active management of the third stage of labor (AMTSL). Traditionally, AMTSL consists of 3 interventions: administration of a uterotonic agent, immediate umbilical cord clamping, and controlled umbilical cord traction to facilitate placenta delivery. The relative importance of each respective component of AMTSL has recently been questioned. For example, a recent randomized trial found that controlled cord traction contributed minimally to controlling blood loss in resource-rich settings if oxytocin was administered.[26] Furthermore, emerging evidence has suggested a neonatal benefit of delayed cord clamping; thus, the primary focus of current research has focused on the type, dose, and timing of the uterotonic agent given.

More than 30 randomized trials have compared various doses of medications, including oxytocin, oxytocin/ergometrine (Syntometrine), prostaglandins (misoprostol, carboprost, dinoprostone), carbetocin (oxytocin analogue), and tranexamic acid in the setting of vaginal or cesarean delivery. The most commonly used and most readily available medication for postpartum hemorrhage prevention regardless of delivery mode remains oxytocin, with traditional dosing 10 to 40 U in 1 L intravenously (IV) over 4 to 6 hours.[17,27]

One promising newer agent for postpartum hemorrhage prevention in the setting of cesarean delivery is tranexamic acid, an antifibrinolytic amino acid derivative of lysine. A recent systematic review and meta-analysis of 9 randomized controlled trials (RCTs) demonstrated significant decreased blood loss compared with standard prophylactic oxytocin.[28] Despite these positive findings in 2365 women in 9 RCTs, the authors recommend further investigation to assess the effect of this medication on thromboembolic events and mortality.

Table 2
Summary of postpartum hemorrhage diagnosis, incidence, risk factors, and management

	Comments	References
Diagnosis	• Cumulative blood loss of >1000 mL OR blood loss accompanied by sign/symptoms of hypovolemia within 24 h following the birth process • Blood loss of 500 mL or more within 24 h after birth	American Congress of Obstetricians and Gynecologists,[19] California Maternal Quality Care Collaborative[20] World Health Organization[21]
Incidence	• 4%–6% of all pregnancies • 3 of 1000 experience severe hemorrhage (blood transfusion, hysterectomy and/or surgical repair of uterus)	American Congress of Obstetricians and Gynecologists,[23] 2006; Kramer et al,[24] 2013; Royal College of Obstetricians and Gynecologists[25]

Risk factors	• Preexisting factors
	  ○ History of postpartum hemorrhage
	  ○ Preeclampsia
	  ○ Overdistended uterus (macrosomia, twins, hydramnios)
	  ○ Obesity
	  ○ Anemia
	  ○ Asian or Hispanic ethnicity
	• Antepartum factors
	  ○ Prolonged, augmented or rapid labor
	  ○ Episiotomy
	  ○ Operative delivery
	  ○ Infection
	  ○ Induction of labor
	• Placental factors
	  ○ Abruption
	  ○ Previa
	  ○ Retained placenta
	  ○ Abnormal placentation
		American Congress of Obstetricians and Gynecologists,[23] 2006; Royal College of Obstetricians and Gynecologists[25]

Treatment (Management)	• Medical management	Dahlke et al,[17] 2015; American Congress of Obstetricians and Gynecologists,[23] 2006; Royal College of Obstetricians and Gynecologists[25]
	○ Oxytocin 10–40 U IV or 10 U IM	
	○ Methylergonovine (Methedrine) 0.2 mg IM every 2–4 h	
	○ PDF2α (Hemabate) 0.25 mg IM every 15–20 min, 8 dose maximum	
	○ PGE1 (misoprostol) 800–1000 mcg rectal	
	○ Carbetocin 100 mcg IV over 1 min	
	○ Tranexamic acid 10 mg/kg 10–20 min before surgery	
	• Surgical management	
	• Uterine packing 4-in gauze, 5000 U thrombin in 5 mL saline	
	• Balloon tamponade 300–800 mL saline based on manufacturer	
	• Brace suture	
	○ B-Lynch	
	○ Square	
	• Vessel ligation	
	○ Uterine artery	
	○ Internal iliac	
	• Hysterectomy	
	• Radiologic embolization	

Abbreviations: IM, intramuscularly; PGE1, prostaglandin E1; PGF2α, prostaglandin-F2α.

Management

A variety of tools are available to the clinician to manage postpartum hemorrhage, including medication, surgical interventions, and radiologic embolization procedures. There are no randomized trials that have established the order for which each intervention should occur; but generally, the least invasive intervention should precede a more invasive one. National guidelines from the ACOG and RCOG vary with regard to the optimal management of postpartum hemorrhage.[23,25] Both guidelines do, however, recommend each institution establish a policy or protocol for how postpartum hemorrhage is identified and treated. One such algorithm that can serve as a template for a protocol if one does not exist is included in the CMQCC's obstetric hemorrhage toolkit.[20] Although certainly beneficial to the clinicians and institutions, it must be stated that these initiatives have yet to be prospectively evaluated with regard to improving postpartum hemorrhage outcomes.[17]

Table 2 summarizes the most common medications available to treat ongoing postpartum hemorrhage. It is important to recognize that the primary mechanism of action of these medications involves improving uterine tone. Although this may help resolve most causes of postpartum hemorrhage, less common causes, such as trauma or coagulopathy, must always be considered, especially if the hemorrhage is not responsive to initial medical management.

Surgical options include tamponade procedures, such as uterine packing, and more recently balloon tamponade devices. These interventions may require a learning curve on the part of the clinician to implement correctly if he or she is unfamiliar with them. In addition, although balloon tamponade devices have been incorporated into various protocols and algorithms, none have been compared with any other treatment strategy in an RCT.[29]

Surgical treatment options, including brace sutures, such as the B-lynch or square suture; vessel ligation (uterine or internal iliac); and hysterectomy, require the ability to perform a laparotomy and a surgeon experienced in the various techniques. Given the rarity of hemorrhage that requires this type of treatment, coordination with subspecialists and surgeons experienced with these techniques is paramount. Highlighting this importance is a recent survey of French obstetricians that found almost 1 in 5 respondents who did not have mastery of any of the surgical techniques for postpartum hemorrhage management.[30]

Finally, when the aforementioned surgical interventions are required, intensive resuscitative efforts are often occurring concurrently. Communication between anesthesia providers and the surgical team remains paramount. Surgeons should clearly communicate the state of ongoing bleeding and the interventions anticipated. Anesthesia can also clearly communicate both the stability of patients along with current and anticipated blood product use. One well-established method to facilitate this communication and maximize blood product availability includes incorporation of massive transfusion protocols into management protocols.

Massive transfusion protocols emphasize early utilization of blood products, and it is currently the preferred method of resuscitative efforts.[31]

SUMMARY

Shoulder dystocia and postpartum hemorrhage represent two of the most common emergencies faced in obstetric clinical practice, both requiring prompt recognition and management in order to avoid significant morbidity or mortality. Shoulder dystocia is an uncommon, unpredictable, and unpreventable obstetric situation occurring in approximately 0.6% to 1.4% of all deliveries and can be managed with appropriate interventions, including initial maneuvers, such as McRoberts and suprapubic pressure; internal maneuvers, such as anterior or posterior shoulder rotation; or third-line maneuvers, including Zavanelli, cleidotomy, and symphysiotomy. Postpartum hemorrhage occurs more commonly, in 4% to 6% of all deliveries, and carries significant risk of maternal morbidity. Postpartum hemorrhage prophylaxis, such as the AMTSL, is well established. An understanding of the medical, surgical, and radiologic treatment options available to the clinician is necessary. The first step in addressing both obstetric emergencies involves effective communication of the clinical scenario in order to appropriate the correct resources. Institutional protocols and algorithms for the prevention and management of both shoulder dystocia and postpartum hemorrhage are becoming increasingly more common and can provide invaluable resources for delivering providers. In summary, shoulder dystocia and postpartum hemorrhage will undoubtedly be experienced by obstetric providers; knowledge of its cause, preventative strategies, and management options is paramount.

REFERENCES

1. American College of Obstetricians and Gynecologists. ACOG practice bulletin no 40: shoulder dystocia. Washington, DC: The College; 2002. Reaffirmed 2015. Available at: http://www.acog.org/Resources-And-Publications/Practice-Bulletins/Committee-on-Practice-Bulletins-Obstetrics/Shoulder-Dystocia. Accessed July 15, 2016.
2. Spong CY, Beall M, Rodrigues D, et al. An objective definition of shoulder dystocia: prolonged head-to-body delivery intervals and/or the use of ancillary obstetric maneuvers. Obstet Gynecol 1995;86:433–6.
3. Royal College of Obstetricians and Gynaecologists. Green top guidelines. London: RCOG; 2012. Available at: https://www.rcog.org.uk/globalassets/documents/guidelines/gtg_42.pdf. Accessed July 15, 2016.
4. Chauhan SP, Gherman R, Hendrix NW, et al. Shoulder dystocia: comparison of the ACOG practice bulletin with another national guideline. Am J Perinatol 2010;27:129–36.
5. Hansen A, Chauhan SP. Shoulder dystocia: definitions and incidence. Semin Perinatol 2014;38:184–8.
6. Bingham J, Chauhan SP, Hayes E, et al. Recurrent shoulder dystocia: a review. Obstet Gynecol Surv 2010;65:183–8.
7. Gross TL, Sokol RJ, Williams T, et al. Shoulder dystocia: a fetal-physician risk. Am J Obstet Gynecol 1987;156:1408–18.
8. American College of Obstetricians and Gynecologists; Society for Maternal-Fetal Medicine. Obstetric care consensus no. 1: safe prevention of the primary cesarean delivery. Obstet Gynecol 2014;123:693–711.
9. Chauhan SP, Hendrix NW, Magann EF, et al. A review of sonographic estimate of fetal weight: vagaries of accuracy. J Matern Fetal Neonatal Med 2005;18:211–20.
10. Chauhan SP, Blackwell SB, Ananth CV. Neonatal brachial plexus palsy: incidence, prevalence, and temporal trends. Semin Perinatol 2014;38:210–8.
11. Grobman WA, Miller D, Burke C, et al. Outcomes associated with introduction of a shoulder dystocia protocol. Am J Obstet Gynecol 2011;205:513–7.
12. Hoffman MK, Bailit JL, Branch DW, et al, Consortium on Safe Labor. A comparison of obstetric maneuvers for the acute management of shoulder dystocia. Obstet Gynecol 2011;117:1272–8.
13. Chauhan SP, Laye MR, Lutgendorf M, et al. A multicenter assessment of 1,177 cases of shoulder dystocia: lessons learned. Am J Perinatol 2014;31:401–6.

14. Bruner JP, Drummond SB, Meenan AL, et al. All-fours maneuver for reducing shoulder dystocia during labor. J Reprod Med 1998;43:439–43.

15. Chauhan SP. Shoulder dystocia and neonatal brachial plexus palsy: eliminating the nightmare. Semin Perinatol 2014;38:183.

16. Chang KW, Ankumah NA, Wilson TJ, et al. Persistence of neonatal brachial plexus palsy associated with maternally reported route of delivery: review of 387 cases. Am J Perinatol 2016;33:765–9.

17. Dahlke JD, Mendez-Figueroa H, Maggio L, et al. Prevention and management of postpartum hemorrhage: a comparison of 4 national guidelines. Am J Obstet Gynecol 2015;213(1):76.e1-10.

18. Patel A, Goudar SS, Geller SE, et al. Drape estimation vs. visual assessment for estimating postpartum hemorrhage. Int J Gynaecol Obstet 2006;93(3):220–4.

19. American Congress of Obstetricians and Gynecologists. reVITALize obstetric data definitions. Available at: http://www.acog.org/-/media/Departments/Patient-Safety-and-Quality-Improvement/2014reVITALizeObstetricDataDefinitionsV10.pdf. Accessed July 15, 2016.

20. California Maternal Quality Care Collaborative. OB hemorrhage toolkit. Available at: https://cmqcc.org/ob_hemorrhage. Accessed July 15, 2016.

21. World Health Organization. WHO recommendations for the prevention and treatment of postpartum haemorrhage. Geneva (Switzerland): World Health Organization; 2012. WHO guidelines approved by the Guidelines Review Committee. Available at: http://www.who.int/reproductivehealth/publications/maternal_perinatal_health/9789241548502/en/. Accessed July 15, 2016.

22. Association of Women's Health, Obstetric and Neonatal Nurses (AWHONN). Practice brief number 1: quantification of blood loss. Available at: http://www.pphproject.org/downloads/awhonn_qbl.pdf. Accessed July 15, 2016.

23. American College of Obstetricians and Gynecologists. ACOG practice bulletin: clinical management guidelines for obstetrician-gynecologists number 76, October 2006: postpartum hemorrhage. Obstet Gynecol 2006;108(4):1039–47 (Reaffirmed 2011).

24. Kramer MS, Berg C, Abenhaim H, et al. Incidence, risk factors, and temporal trends in severe postpartum hemorrhage. Am J Obstet Gynecol 2013;209(5):449.e1-7.

25. Royal College of Obstetrician and Gynaecologists. Postpartum hemorrhage: prevention and management. 2011. Available at: http://www.rcog.org.uk/womens-health/clinical-guidance/prevention-and-management-postpartum-haemorrhage-green-top-52. Accessed July 15, 2016.

26. Deneux-Tharaux C, Sentilhes L, Maillard F, et al. Effect of routine controlled cord traction as part of the active management of the third stage of labour on postpartum haemorrhage: multicentre randomised controlled trial (TRACOR). BMJ 2013;346:f1541.

27. Dahlke JD, Mendez-Figueroa H, Rouse DJ, et al. Evidence-based surgery for cesarean delivery: an updated systematic review. Am J Obstet Gynecol 2013;209(4):294–306.

28. Simonazzi G, Bisulli M, Saccone G, et al. Tranexamic acid for preventing postpartum blood loss after cesarean delivery: a systematic review and meta-analysis of randomized controlled trials. Acta Obstet Gynecol Scand 2016;95(1):28–37.

29. Wright CE, Chauhan SP, Abuhamad AZ. Bakri balloon in the management of postpartum hemorrhage: a review. Am J Perinatol 2014;31(11):957–64.

30. Bouet PE, Brun S, Madar H, et al. Surgical management of postpartum haemor-rhage: survey of French obstetricians. Sci Rep 2016;6:30342.
31. Pacheco LD, Saade GR, Costantine MM, et al. An update on the use of massive transfusion protocols in obstetrics. Am J Obstet Gynecol 2016;214(3):340–4.

Prenatal Diagnosis
Screening and Diagnostic Tools

Laura M. Carlson, MD*, Neeta L. Vora, MD

KEYWORDS

- Aneuploidy • Genetic screening • Noninvasive prenatal screening • Cell-free DNA
- Chorionic villus sampling • Amniocentesis

KEY POINTS

- Aneuploidy screening should be offered to all women at their first prenatal visit.
- Cell-free fetal DNA screening is currently recommended for high-risk populations only and should be considered a screening test rather than a diagnostic test.
- Chorionic villus sampling and amniocentesis carry a small but potential risk of pregnancy loss but remain the only diagnostic methodologies available presently.
- Women should receive thorough pretest counseling regarding the risks and benefits of available options and should receive thorough posttest counseling with individualized interpretation of results.

INTRODUCTION

Approximately 3% to 5% of pregnancies are complicated by birth defects or genetic disorders.[1] Chromosomal abnormalities are present in approximately 1 in 150 live births,[2] and congenital malformations remain the leading cause of infant death and a leading cause of childhood death.[3] These chromosomal abnormalities include aneuploidy (defined as having one or more extra or missing chromosomes), translocations, duplications, and deletions.

The most common chromosomal disorder is trisomy 21 (Down syndrome), with an incidence of 1 per 800 live births.[4] Trisomy 13 and 18 can also result in live births, though with a significantly lower incidence.[2,4] Sex chromosome aneuploidies are less common than autosomal aneuploidies.[4] The only known viable monosomy is monosomy X (Turner syndrome). Incidences are described in **Table 1**.

Disclosure: The authors have no conflicts of interest to report.
Division of Maternal Fetal Medicine, Department of Obstetrics and Gynecology, University of North Carolina School of Medicine, 3010 Old Clinic Building, CB #7516, Chapel Hill, NC 27599-7516, USA
* Corresponding author.
E-mail address: laura_carlson@med.unc.edu

Table 1	
Incidence of common aneuploidies	
Trisomy 21	1 in 800 live births
Trisomy 18	1 in 7500 live births
Trisomy 13	1 in 15,000 live births
Monosomy X (Turner syndrome)	1 in 5000 girls
Trisomy X	1 in 1000 girls
XXY (Klinefelter syndrome)	1 in 1000 boys
XYY	1 in 1000 boys

Data from Nussbaum RL, McInnes RR, Willard HF. Thompson & Thompson genetics in medicine. 7th edition. Philadelphia: Saunders/Elsevier; 2007.

Risk of aneuploidy increases with maternal age (**Table 2**).[2,4] Other factors also influence patients' risk in any given pregnancy, including the presence of birth defects or soft markers on ultrasound and past obstetric history, particularly if it is notable for a prior pregnancy affected by aneuploidy or another genetic disorder. A past family history of aneuploidy increases current pregnancy risk of aneuploidy, especially if a parent is a balanced robertsonian translocation carrier, though most cases are sporadic and secondary to chromosomal nondisjunction.

Patients report many different motivations for pursuing aneuploidy screening or prenatal diagnosis. Some may choose pregnancy termination if the defect is identified at an early enough gestational age. Others may choose to pursue screening or testing to allow them time to process the diagnosis and seek experienced clinicians who may be able to aid them in preparation for caring for an affected infant and to care for their child after delivery. Some birth defects, such as some neural tube defects, may be eligible for prenatal treatment with subsequently improved neonatal outcomes.[5] All patients choosing to undergo screening or testing should receive counseling regarding risks, benefits, and limitations of their chosen testing plan from their health care provider or genetic counselor. It is important to note that aneuploidy screening and testing decisions are heavily value driven; a frank discussion of the benefits, risks, and limitations of tests is key in ensuring that care is appropriate for each patient's individual goals.

Table 2		
Risk of aneuploidy by maternal age		
Maternal Age at EDD (y)	**Risk of Trisomy 21**	**Risk of Other Chromosomal Abnormality**
20	1:1480	1:525
25	1:1340	1:475
30	1:940	1:384
35	1:353	1:178
40	1:85	1:62
45	1:35	1:18

Abbreviation: EDD, estimated date of delivery.
Adapted from Practice bulletin no. 163: screening for fetal aneuploidy. Obstet Gynecol 2016;127(5):e124.

HISTORY OF SCREENING

Initial screening for birth defects was developed in the 1950s with ultrasound and has become increasingly prominent in obstetric care. Real-time gray-scale imaging became available in the 1970s and improved prenatal diagnosis by allowing for evaluation of pregnancies earlier in gestation. Aims of ultrasonography include determination of gestational age and fetal number, evaluation for malformations, testing of fetal well-being, and assistance with invasive diagnostic and therapeutic procedures.[6] Amniocentesis, the first available prenatal chromosomal diagnostic testing option, was first described in the 1950s.[7] Amniocentesis has become increasingly safe and is now used for several purposes, including genetic screening and infectious evaluations. Chorionic villus sampling (CVS) is another diagnostic test and can be performed earlier in gestation.

Subsequently, noninvasive tests, including serum analyte screening and cell-free DNA screening, were developed for purposes of screening for genetic abnormalities within a pregnancy.

In 2007, the American Congress of Obstetricians and Gynecologists (ACOG) released "ACOG Practice Bulletin No. 77," which recommended making aneuploidy screening or invasive testing available for all women, ideally at their first prenatal visit.[8] This idea was revolutionary at the time, as previously only women who were considered to be at high risk had been offered these tests.

SCREENING TESTS

Most prenatal testing is intended for screening. These tests include serum screening, carrier screening, and ultrasound; the goals of these tests are to identify women with pregnancies at high risk of chromosomal abnormalities or birth defects. Although ultrasound can be diagnostic, such as in the case of open neural tube defect, serum screening is intended only to identify women with pregnancies at an increased risk. Numerous options for serum screening are available with varying test criteria and timing of employment (**Table 3**).[4]

FIRST-TRIMESTER SCREEN

The first-trimester screen is a commonly used screening test that includes a combination of serum screening and ultrasonographic examination of the nuchal translucency performed between 10 and 13 weeks 6 days' gestation. Serum markers, including free beta–human chorionic gonadotropin (hCG) and pregnancy-associated plasma protein A, are collected with a capillary blood sample between 9 and 13 weeks 6 days' gestation. A risk estimate is then developed that incorporates maternal age, past pregnancy history, number of fetuses in the current gestation, weight, race, serum markers, and nuchal translucency measurement. Some risk estimators also incorporate presence or absence of visualized nasal bone. This risk estimate is then expressed as a ratio, such as 1 in 10. One in 300 is commonly used as the cutoff for a high-risk result, but the cutoff is laboratory dependent. The detection rate for trisomy 21 varies from 82% to 87% depending on the laboratory, using a 5% screen positive rate.[4]

A nuchal translucency of greater than 3 mm is significantly associated with both aneuploidy and structural malformations.[4,9–12] In the initial observational study describing this phenomenon, 35% of patients with a nuchal translucency measurement greater than 3 mm subsequently had confirmed aneuploidy.[9] A subsequent observational study confirmed increased prevalence of cardiac defects in patients with a nuchal translucency greater than 3.5 mm with chromosomally normal

Table 3
Characteristics of serum screening options for aneuploidy

Screening Test	Gestational Age at Screening (in wk)	Detection Rate for Trisomy 21 (%)	Screen Positive Rate (%)	Analytes and/or Measurements Obtained
First-trimester screen	10–13*	82–87[15]	5	Nuchal translucency Papp-A hCG
Triple screen	15–22	69	5	hCG AFP uE3
Quad screen	15–22	81	5	hCG AFP uE3 DIA
Integrated	10–13 and 15–22	96	5	First-trimester screen, then quad screen
Sequential stepwise	10–13 and 15–22	95	5	First-trimester screen, then quad screen
Contingent screen	10–13 and 15–22	88–94	5	First-trimester screen, then quad screen
Cell-free DNA	Any age after 9 10 wk	99	0.5	Molecular evaluation of cell-free fetal DNA within maternal serum

Abbreviations: AFP, alpha-fetoprotein; DIA, dimeric inhibin-A; hCG, human chorionic gonadotropin; Papp-A, pregnancy-associated plasma protein A; uE3, unconjugated estriol.
    * Detection rate varies with gestational age, with improved detection at lower gestational ages.
    Adapted from Practice bulletin no. 163: screening for fetal aneuploidy. Obstet Gynecol 2016;127(5):e126.

pregnancies.[13] Risk of other anomalies, including single gene defects and central nervous system, cardiac, skeletal, and abdominal wall defects, is also significantly increased in these pregnancies.[10] It is, therefore, recommended that any woman with a thickened nuchal translucency undergo a targeted ultrasound and be offered a fetal echocardiogram to assess for presence of other structural cardiac malformations regardless of whether aneuploidy is present or absent.[4]

Benefits of first-trimester screening include the early gestational age at which results are provided, allowing patients and providers time to interpret results and make decisions surrounding further pregnancy care, including pursuit of further diagnostic testing, genetic counseling, maternal fetal medicine consultation, or termination if desired. There are several drawbacks to this screen as well. This test relies on the availability of certified, experienced sonographers to perform the nuchal translucency measurement. It has been previously demonstrated that a measurement discrepancy of only 0.5 mm significantly decreases the sensitivity of this test.[14] The test's improved sensitivity over the quadruple marker screen also varies with gestational age; the test has improved detection at 11 weeks, though performance characteristics are similar to the quadruple marker screen at 13 weeks.[15]

QUADRUPLE MARKER SCREEN

The quadruple marker screen, or the quad screen, is the initial serum screening test that became available in the 1990s. It is still commonly used today, particularly in patients who present for care after the first trimester, which comprises more than 25% of patients using public health clinics.[16] The quad screen may be performed between 15 and 22 weeks' gestation and involves serum measurements of proteins secreted by the pregnancy, including hCG, alpha-fetoprotein (AFP), inhibin A, and unconjugated estriol. These protein measurements are combined with the patients' age, race, weight, number of fetuses in the current gestation, diabetes status, and gestational age to provide a risk estimate. Detection rate is slightly lower than that of the first-trimester screen, with a reported detection rate of 81% using a 5% screen positive rate.[4]

Advantages of the quad screen include its ability to screen for open neural tube defects in addition to aneuploidy. Serum AFP is secreted by the fetus and is present in the amniotic fluid and, therefore, also maternal serum. It also does not require a specially trained sonographer to perform and, thus, may be more readily available to some providers.

Several centers may offer variations on the quad screen, including the triple screen, which does not include inhibin measurements,[17] or the penta screen, which also includes hyperglycosylated hCG.[18] These tests do not seem to have improved test characteristics.

INTEGRATED, STEPWISE SEQUENTIAL, AND CONTINGENT SCREENING

Numerous screening modalities incorporate both a first-trimester screen and the quad screen. These modalities included integrated screening, the stepwise sequential screen, and the contingent screening. Integrated screening involves performing a first trimester screen, of which the results are not providing to the patient or provider, and subsequently performing a quad screen. All of these values are then incorporated into a single risk estimate to provide patient a comprehensive risk of her second trimester risk of aneuploidy. The detection rate is 96%, the highest of any available serum screens other than cell-free DNA, with a 5% screen positive rate. Downsides to this approach include its relatively late availability of results, limiting the time in which patients and their provider may have to make important decisions about future care.

Both the stepwise sequential screen and the contingent screen make first-trimester screening results available to patients. The stepwise sequential screen involves performing the first-trimester screen and the quad screen. Results are available to women after their first-trimester screen, allowing for earlier counseling and diagnosis for patients at high risk of aneuploidy. The contingent screen involves performing a first-trimester screen for all women, after which women are stratified into high-, medium-, and low-risk groups. The high-risk group is then offered a diagnostic test. The low-risk group has no further testing. The intermediate-risk group is offered quad screening. The detection rate varies between 80% and 94% for this screening method, with a 5% screen positive rate.

CELL-FREE FETAL DNA

Cell-free DNA, commonly referred to as noninvasive prenatal screening, became commercially available in 2011. This relatively new technology involves collecting a maternal serum sample, from which cell-free fragments of DNA from the pregnancy are isolated. This cell-free DNA is primarily placental in origin and is released from apoptotic trophoblasts. Fetal fraction increases with gestational age but is reliably greater than 10% as early as 10 weeks' gestation. Notably, fetal fraction of greater than 4% is required for reliable analysis. This cell-free DNA is then evaluated by one of 2 techniques (via massive parallel shotgun sequencing, targeted massive parallel sequencing, or interrogation of single nucleotide polymorphisms),[19] depending on which laboratory is running the analysis. Results are typically reported with aneuploidy detected or no aneuploidy detected or as high- or low-risk for aneuploidy and with sex chromosome information if desired.

This screening test has the highest available detection rate of all available screening tests for trisomy 21 with a detection rate of 99% on a recently updated meta-analysis.[20] Detection rates for trisomy 18, 13, and sex chromosome abnormalities are significantly lower than for trisomy 21 (**Table 4**).[20] It is important to note that at present, cell-free DNA for aneuploidy screening is only recommended by the ACOG for women with high pretest risk of aneuploidy, as described in **Box 1**. It is also notable that the studies that provided the test characteristics described earlier excluded patients who did not have sufficient fetal fraction to provide a risk estimate. It has subsequently been found that an inconclusive result significantly increases aneuploidy risk, with low fetal fraction significantly associated with aneuploidy, particularly trisomy 13 and 18.[21] Other factors that may influence fetal fraction include weight, with obese women having an increased risk of low fetal fraction, and lower gestational age.[21,22]

This test should be clearly conveyed to patients as a screening test rather than a diagnostic test. The positive predictive value for trisomy 21 in the population for whom it is currently recommended is very high. However, positive predictive value depends on the prevalence of the disorder within the population. Therefore, the positive predictive value is expected to be significantly lower in an average-risk population. A recent retrospective cohort study out of 2 academic centers identified 105 patients with cell-free DNA results consistent with autosomal trisomies; of these, aneuploidy was only confirmed in 82% by karyotype, with the remainder of patients having normal antenatal or postnatal karyotype.[23] Previous studies have shown that patients' misunderstanding of this test is significant despite pretest counseling.[24] Notably, in the aforementioned cohort, 9 patients underwent termination of pregnancy without diagnostic confirmation of a chromosomal abnormality.[23] Any results should be interpreted with the aid of a genetic counselor in order to provide further guidance as to patients' individual risk. Calculators for individual risk estimates using cell-free DNA results are available through both the University of North Carolina's MomBaby Web site (available at med.unc.edu/obgyn/Patient_Care/specialty-services/maternal-fetal medicine/mombaby/nips_calc.html; retrieved July 22, 2016) and the Perinatal Quality Foundation (available at perinatalquality.org; retrieved July 22, 2016). Ultrasound is recommended before testing to confirm fetal number and gestational age and to

Table 4
Estimated detection rate of cell-free DNA for aneuploidy and positive predictive value by maternal age

	Pooled Detection Rate[20] (%)	PPV at 25 y of Age[a] (%)	PPV at 35 y of Age[a] (%)	PPV at 45 y of Age[a] (%)
Trisomy 21	99.2	51	79	98
Trisomy 18	96.3	15	39	90
Trisomy 13	91.7	7	21	Data insufficient to calculate
Monosomy X	90.3	41	41	41

Abbreviation: PPV, positive predictive value.
[a] Predictive values calculated via the Perinatal Quality Foundation calculator. Available at perinatalquality.org; retrieved July 22, 2016.

Box 1
Indications for cell-free DNA screening

- Maternal age greater than 35 years at delivery
- Ultrasonographic findings indicating increased aneuploidy risk
- History of prior pregnancy affected by a trisomy
- Parental balanced robertsonian translocation increasing risk of trisomy 13 or 21
- High-risk first-trimester or second-trimester aneuploidy screening results

Data from Cell-free DNA screening for fetal aneuploidy. Committee Opinion No. 640. American College of Obstetricians and Gynecologists. Obstet Gynecol 2015;126(3):e31–7.

---

evaluate for presence of major anomalies identifiable in the first trimester, as this would alter a priori aneuploidy risk. In one retrospective cohort, 16% of patients were found to have ultrasound findings that altered counseling and recommendations regarding testing or screening modality, including incorrect pregnancy dating, embryonic or fetal demise, twin gestation or presence of an anomaly.[25] In those cases in which a cystic hygroma or anomaly is identified, patients may choose to undergo diagnostic testing rather than screening, allowing for earlier prenatal diagnosis.[25]

Other benefits of cell-free DNA include its ability to accurately identify fetal sex with excellent accuracy and fetal Rh status in pregnancies at risk of Rh isoimmunization.[26] Food and Drug Administration–approved cell-free DNA technology for anti-Kell and other sources of isoimmunization is not yet available in the United States. Several laboratories have begun to report on other autosomal aneuploidies or for microdeletions; however, these tests are not currently validated and are not recommended at present.[4,27] In fact, a retrospective analysis evaluating a small number of cases yielded 0% positive predictive values for evaluated microdeletions; given low prevalence of microdeletion syndromes, positive predictive value for most microdeletions is not expected to surpass 10%.[28] Use of cell-free DNA has also not been widely studied in multiple gestations, and use is currently not recommended in this setting.[27]

It is also worth noting that occasionally, cell-free DNA screening will reveal maternal chromosomal abnormalities or concerns, including maternal mosaicism or, rarely, maternal malignancies.[29] Patients should be counseled of this possibility before proceeding with screening. Maternal chromosomal abnormalities or malignancy may result in nonreportable or false-positive results. Other possible sources of false-positive results include vanishing twins or confined placental mosaicism. It is also worth noting that although cell-free DNA has the best detection rate for trisomy 21 of any screening modalities, sequential screening continues to have an improved detection rate for all chromosomal abnormalities over cell-free DNA, indicating that many other chromosomal abnormalities that may be identified with traditional serum screening may be missed with cell-free DNA.[30]

ULTRASOUND ONLY

Ultrasound is now ubiquitous in pregnancy management. Nearly all women receive at least one ultrasonographic examination of their pregnancy during a routine obstetric care, and many receive more than one. The primary function of ultrasound and obstetric care is for confirmation of dating as well as surveillance for birth defects.

Many patients choose to pursue ultrasound screening only for evaluation of malformations or markers for aneuploidy, as second-trimester transabdominal ultrasonography performed between 18 and 23 weeks has become routine in prenatal care to evaluate for anatomic anomalies. Many patients also undergo first-trimester ultrasonography via either a transvaginal or transabdominal route to evaluate for viability, pregnancy number, and for evaluation of major anomalies that can be identified in the first trimester, such as anencephaly or cystic hygromas. Some anomalies have known associations with particular aneuploidies or chromosomal defects, increasing the likelihood of the presence of these conditions when identified.

DIAGNOSTIC TESTING

Diagnostic testing allows patients to know with as much certainty as possible whether their pregnancy may be affected by a particular genetic condition. The most common indication for diagnostic testing in the United States currently is advanced maternal age or maternal age of 35 years or older on the estimated date of delivery. Other common indications include positive aneuploidy screening results, known family history of genetic disorders, or anomalies identified on ultrasound. Although diagnostic testing is recommended by the ACOG to be available to all women, regardless of maternal age, patients should be counseled before proceeding on risk of pregnancy loss.

CHORIONIC VILLUS SAMPLING

CVS has decreased in frequency with the recent increased uptake of cell-free DNA screening. It remains the only diagnostic test available in the first trimester and allows for diagnostic analyses, including fluorescence in situ hybridization (FISH), karyotype, microarray, molecular testing, and gene sequencing. CVS is performed between 10 and 14 weeks' gestation. CVS has been performed before 9 weeks in the past, though this has shown to increase the risk of limb deformities and, therefore, is no longer recommended.

CVS may be performed via either transcervical or transabdominal approach. Via either approach, chorionic villi are collected for genetic evaluation under ultrasound guidance without entering the amniotic sac. CVS allows for earlier prenatal diagnosis, subsequently decreasing time of uncertainty and allowing for earlier (and, therefore, safer) pregnancy termination if desired. A disadvantage of CVS, however, is that approximately 1% to 2% of CVS results may reflect confined placental mosaicism rather than true fetal chromosomal abnormalities. Confined placental mosaicism may increase the risk of having a small-for-gestational-age infant.[31] Pregnancy loss attributed to CVS is approximately 1 in 455 on the most recent estimates.[32,33]

AMNIOCENTESIS

Amniocentesis, similar to CVS, has decreased in frequency with increased utilization of cell-free fetal DNA screening. It remains the only diagnostic test available in the second or third trimesters of pregnancy and may be performed at any gestational age after 15 weeks. Using this technique, a sterile needle is introduced into the amniotic sac under ultrasound guidance, and amniotic fluid is obtained and sent for testing. In addition to evaluation for genetic disorders, amniocentesis may also be used to evaluate for presence of intra-amniotic or fetal infection via culture or polymerase chain reaction or for neural tube defects by measuring amniotic fluid alpha-fetoprotein and acetylcholinesterase. Complications are more common at earlier gestational ages. Pregnancy loss attributed to amniocentesis is approximately 1 in 900 on most recent estimates.[32,33]

CYTOGENETIC EVALUATIONS

Chromosome analysis from CVS and amniocentesis samples is the most reliably predictive method of identifying pregnancies affected by chromosomal disorders. However, some issues with cytogenetic testing have been identified that may limit the clinical utility of these methods.

Mosaicism refers to tissue that contains 2 or more distinct cell lines. It is thought to reflect true mosaicism when multiple colonies from multiple cultures reveal the same results. Pseudomosaicism refers to a single cell with a different genetic makeup than the others and is usually not clinically significant. Mosaicism may also arise in primary cell culture; when this occurs, it reflects pseudomosaicism rather than true mosaicism. Particular to CVS, confined placental mosaicism occurs in approximately 1% to 2% of pregnancies; although this does reflect true mosaicism, it carries different clinical concerns for the fetus than for other pregnancies. As confined placental mosaicism also causes false-positive cell-free DNA results, amniocentesis is preferred over CVS for diagnostic testing in cases of positive cell-free DNA. With some trisomies, particularly trisomy 15, a diploid fetus often arises secondary to trisomy rescue, which does increase the risk of uniparental disomy and subsequently increases risk of Prader-Willi and Angelman syndrome. Cell culture failure also rarely occurs and is more common with sampling via CVS than with amniocentesis.

Multiple testing methodologies are available, designed to detect different types of genetic abnormalities. Large deletions and duplications may be identified with karyotype in more than 5 million base pairs, whereas small deletions and duplications may be identified with microarray technology at as small as a 50,000 base pair level.[34] FISH technology is available for identification of major autosomal aneuploidies or for selected deletions and duplications, such as DiGeorge syndrome. Single-gene disorders often require more targeted molecular approach to identify whether or not a particular mutation in a particular panel of genes is present or absent. As detection of aneuploidy is the most common indication for invasive testing, FISH is often the first test that is sent. This technology does not require cell culture; thus, results are often available within 48 hours. Despite that these results are obtained from a diagnostic procedure, these results should still be considered a screen and should be confirmed via karyotype given rare reports of both false-positive and false-negative results.[35] Microarray can also be performed on uncultured cells and, therefore, can also result in a more rapid turnaround time. Results can also be obtained from nonviable cells with this technique and, thus, may be more likely to result in cases of stillbirth. Given that microarray is able to detect both aneuploidy and smaller deletions and duplications with rapid turnaround, it is now recommended for evaluation of structural abnormalities as the initial testing strategy along with FISH, rather than conventional karyotype.[33]

As availability and uptake of cytogenetic testing with microarray increases, increasing numbers of chromosomal abnormalities without known clinical consequences have been identified, which may increase parental anxiety when one of these variants of uncertain significance is identified. In these cases, parental studies are often considered to determine whether the variant is present in either parent. If so, it is more likely to be of little to no clinical significance. Given that 1.7% of structurally normal pregnancies without aneuploidy will have a variant of unknown significance detected,[36] patients opting for an amniocentesis with a normal anatomic survey should be counseled about the possibility of the finding of a variant of uncertain clinical significance with microarray testing.[33]

PREIMPLANTATION GENETIC DIAGNOSIS

Preimplantation genetic diagnosis (PGD) is now widely available and may allow for even earlier detection of chromosomal abnormalities. This procedure is performed after in vitro fertilization (IVF) by manipulation of the embryo to either remove a polar body or to remove a single cell from the blastocyst. This procedure allows for detection of the abnormality before embryo transfer so that only unaffected embryos are transferred back. It is recommended that all pregnancies conceived with IVF/PGD be offered confirmatory testing with CVS or amniocentesis as false-negative reports are possible[37] with an anticipated negative predictive value of normal FISH of 81%.[38] The growing body of literature surrounding PGD illustrates minimal risk outside of the cost of this procedure.[33]

SUMMARY

All women should be offered aneuploidy screening or diagnostic testing during pregnancy. Just as importantly, available options should be explained to patients and families in depth, most notably including the risks and benefits of each option, and how results might be reported. Patients who choose cell-free fetal DNA technology should be counseled that the test remains a screening test for aneuploidy at this time and that microdeletion testing continues to have poor positive predictive values due to the low prevalence of these disorders. It is not recommended that patients undergo more than one screening modality but rather that women who have positive screens and wish to pursue further testing be counseled on diagnostic testing with amniocentesis and CVS so as not to delay diagnosis. Amniocentesis and CVS are increasingly safe with low rates of pregnancy loss and should continue to be available to all women who desire diagnostic testing regardless of risk factors or presence or absence of anomalies.

REFERENCES

1. Centers for Disease Control and Prevention (CDC). Update on overall prevalence of major birth defects–Atlanta, Georgia, 1978-2005. MMWR Morb Mortal Wkly Rep 2008;57(1):1–5.
2. Nussbaum RL, McInnes RR, Willard HF, et al. Thompson & Thompson genetics in medicine. 7th edition. Philadelphia: Saunders/Elsevier; 2007.
3. Kochanek KD, Kirmeyer SE, Martin JA, et al. Annual summary of vital statistics: 2009. Pediatrics 2012;129(2):338–48.
4. Practice bulletin No. 163: screening for fetal aneuploidy. Obstet Gynecol 2016; 127(5):e123–37.
5. Adzick NS, Thom EA, Spong CY, et al. A randomized trial of prenatal versus postnatal repair of myelomeningocele. N Engl J Med 2011;364(11):993–1004.
6. Bianchi DW, Bianchi DW. Fetology: diagnosis and management of the fetal patient. 2nd edition. New York: McGraw-Hill Medical Publication Division; 2010.
7. Serr DM, Sachs L, Danon M. The diagnosis of sex before birth using cells from the amniotic fluid (a preliminary report). Bull Res Counc Isr 1955;5B(2):137–8.
8. ACOG Committee on Practice Bulletins. ACOG practice bulletin No. 77: screening for fetal chromosomal abnormalities. Obstet Gynecol 2007;109(1): 217–27.
9. Nicolaides KH, Azar G, Byrne D, et al. Fetal nuchal translucency: ultrasound screening for chromosomal defects in first trimester of pregnancy. BMJ 1992; 304(6831):867–9.

10. Baer RJ, Norton ME, Shaw GM, et al. Risk of selected structural abnormalities in infants after increased nuchal translucency measurement. Am J Obstet Gynecol 2014;211(6):675.e1—19.

11. Galindo A, Comas C, Martinez JM, et al. Cardiac defects in chromosomally normal fetuses with increased nuchal translucency at 10-14 weeks of gestation. J Matern Fetal Neonatal Med 2003;13(3):163-70.

12. Hyett JA, Perdu M, Sharland GK, et al. Increased nuchal translucency at 10-14 weeks of gestation as a marker for major cardiac defects. Ultrasound Obstet Gynecol 1997;10(4):242-6.

13. Hyett J, Noble P, Sebire NJ, et al. Lethal congenital arthrogryposis presents with increased nuchal translucency at 10-14 weeks of gestation. Ultrasound Obstet Gynecol 1997;9(5):310-3.

14. Evans MI, Krantz DA, Hallahan TW, et al. Impact of nuchal translucency credentialing by the FMF, the NTQR or both on screening distributions and performance. Ultrasound Obstet Gynecol 2012;39(2):181-4.

15. Malone FD, Canick JA, Ball RH, et al. First-trimester or second-trimester screening, or both, for Down's syndrome. N Engl J Med 2005;353(19):2001-11.

16. U.S. Department of Health and Human Services HRaSA, Maternal and Child Health Bureau. Child health USA 2013. Rockville (MD): US Department of Health and Human Services; 2013.

17. Conde-Agudelo A, Kafury-Goeta AC. Triple-marker test as screening for Down syndrome: a meta-analysis. Obstet Gynecol Surv 1998;53(6):369-76.

18. Palomaki GE, Neveux LM, Knight GJ, et al. Maternal serum invasive trophoblast antigen (hyperglycosylated hCG) as a screening marker for Down syndrome during the second trimester. Clin Chem 2004;50(10):1804-8.

19. Dar P, Shani H, Evans MI. Cell-free DNA: comparison of technologies. Clin Lab Med 2016;36(2):199-211.

20. Gil MM, Quezada MS, Revello R, et al. Analysis of cell-free DNA in maternal blood in screening for fetal aneuploidies: updated meta-analysis. Ultrasound Obstet Gynecol 2015;45(3):249-66.

21. Suzumori N, Ebara T, Yamada T, et al. Fetal cell-free DNA fraction in maternal plasma is affected by fetal trisomy. J Hum Genet 2016;61(7):647-52.

22. Ashoor G, Syngelaki A, Poon LC, et al. Fetal fraction in maternal plasma cell-free DNA at 11-13 weeks' gestation: relation to maternal and fetal characteristics. Ultrasound Obstet Gynecol 2013;41(1):26-32.

23. Dobson LJ, Reiff ES, Little SE, et al. Patient choice and clinical outcomes following positive noninvasive prenatal screening for aneuploidy with cell-free DNA (cfDNA). Prenat Diagn 2016;36(5):456-62.

24. Piechan JL, Hines KA, Koller DL, et al. NIPT and informed consent: an assessment of patient understanding of a negative NIPT result. J Genet Couns 2016;25(5):1127-37.

25. Vora NL, Robinson S, Hardisty EE, et al. The utility of a prerequisite ultrasound at 10-14 weeks in cell free DNA fetal aneuploidy screening. Ultrasound Obstet Gynecol 2016. [Epub ahead of print].

26. Mackie FL, Hemming K, Allen S, et al. The accuracy of cell-free fetal DNA-based non-invasive prenatal testing in singleton pregnancies: a systematic review and bivariate meta-analysis. BJOG 2016;124(1):32-46.

27. Committee opinion No. 640: cell-free DNA screening for fetal aneuploidy. Obstet Gynecol 2015;126(3):e31-7.

28. Yaron Y, Jani J, Schmid M, et al. Current status of testing for microdeletion syndromes and rare autosomal trisomies using cell-free DNA technology. Obstet Gynecol 2015;126(5):1095–9.

29. Bianchi DW, Chudova D, Sehnert AJ, et al. Noninvasive prenatal testing and incidental detection of occult maternal malignancies. JAMA 2015;314(2):162–9.

30. Norton ME, Baer RJ, Wapner RJ, et al. Cell-free DNA vs sequential screening for the detection of fetal chromosomal abnormalities. Am J Obstet Gynecol 2016; 214(6):727.e1-e6.

31. Baffero GM, Somigliana E, Crovetto F, et al. Confined placental mosaicism at chorionic villous sampling: risk factors and pregnancy outcome. Prenat Diagn 2012; 32(11):1102–8.

32. Akolekar R, Beta J, Picciarelli G, et al. Procedure-related risk of miscarriage following amniocentesis and chorionic villus sampling: a systematic review and meta-analysis. Ultrasound Obstet Gynecol 2015;45(1):16–26.

33. Practice bulletin No. 162: prenatal diagnostic testing for genetic disorders. Obstet Gynecol 2016;127(5):e108–22.

34. Society for Maternal-Fetal M, Dugoff L, Norton ME, et al. The use of chromosomal microarray for prenatal diagnosis. Am J Obstet Gynecol 2016;215(4):B2–9.

35. Tepperberg J, Pettenati MJ, Rao PN, et al. Prenatal diagnosis using interphase fluorescence in situ hybridization (FISH): 2-year multi-center retrospective study and review of the literature. Prenat Diagn 2001;21(4):293–301.

36. Wapner RJ, Martin CL, Levy B, et al. Chromosomal microarray versus karyotyping for prenatal diagnosis. N Engl J Med 2012;367(23):2175–84.

37. Audibert F, Wilson RD, Allen V, et al. Preimplantation genetic testing. J Obstet Gynaecol Can 2009;31(8):761–75.

38. DeUgarte CM, Li M, Surrey M, et al. Accuracy of FISH analysis in predicting chromosomal status in patients undergoing preimplantation genetic diagnosis. Fertil Steril 2008;90(4):1049–54.

Cancer Recognition and Screening for Common Breast Disorders and Malignancy

CrossMark

Constance Bohon, MD

KEYWORDS

• Cancer recognition • Screening • Common breast disorders • Malignancy

KEY POINTS

- Breast cancer is predicted to be the most common newly diagnosed cancer in women in 2016, as it was in 2015.
- Although there is no consensus on optimal strategies, target populations, or the harms and benefits, screening mammography is the most commonly used method for the detection of breast cancer in women of average risk.
- Clinical breast examinations are recommended every 1 to 3 years from age 20 to 39 years and annually beginning at age 40 years by the American College of Obstetricians and Gynecologists (ACOG) and National Comprehensive Cancer Network.
- ACOG recommends a genetic risk assessment for women with a greater than 20% to 25% chance of having an inherited predisposition to breast and ovarian cancer.
- The evaluation of a breast mass begins with a detailed history, assessment for breast cancer risk, and physical examination.

INCIDENCE

Breast cancer is predicted to be the most common newly diagnosed cancer in women in 2016, as it was in 2015. The estimated number of new cases for 2016 is 246,660,[1] with the estimate of 231,840 in 2015.[2] Based on these estimates, breast cancer accounts for 29% of all cancers in women for both years.[1,2] The estimated number of deaths from breast cancer in women also is effectively unchanged, with 40,290 occurring in 2015[2] and 40,450 in 2016.[1]

The probability of developing invasive breast cancer from 2010 to 2012 was 1.9 (1 in 53) for girls and women from birth to age 49 years, 2.3 (1 in 44) for women ages 50 to 59 years, 3.5 (1 in 29) for women aged 60 to 69 years, and 6.7 (1 in 15) for women 70 years of age and older. The overall rate from birth to death was 12.3 (1 in 8).[1]

From 2008 to 2012 the incidence of breast cancer increased in non-Hispanic black (black) and Asian/Pacific Islander women, whereas it was stable in non-Hispanic white

George Washington University School of Medicine and Health Sciences, Washington DC 20037, USA
E-mail address: Constance.Bohon@gmail.com

Obstet Gynecol Clin N Am 44 (2017) 257–270
http://dx.doi.org/10.1016/j.ogc.2017.02.005
0889-8545/17/© 2017 Elsevier Inc. All rights reserved.

obgyn.theclinics.com

(white), Hispanic, and American Indian/Alaska Native (AI/AN) women. Overall, white and black women have a higher incidence and death rate from breast cancer than women of other races/ethnicities. The median age for the diagnosis of breast cancer in women is 61 years, with the median age of 58 years for black women and 62 years for white women. The incidence of breast cancer also varies between states. For example, the incidence of breast cancer among women in Arkansas was 107.7 per 100,000 women, whereas it was 164.4 cases per 100,000 women in Washington, DC among white women. In black women the incidence varied from 94 per 100,000 women in Minnesota to 141.7 per 100,000 women in Alaska.[3]

Based on the Surveillance, Epidemiology and End Results (SEER) program, the incidence of invasive breast cancer decreased by 0.5% from 1975 to 1980, increased by 4% from 1980 to 1987, decreased by 0.2% from 1987 to 1994, increased by 1.8% from 1994 to 1999, decreased by 2.3% from 1999 to 2004, and increased by 0.4% from 2004 to 2013 (**Fig. 1**).[4]

Breast cancer is predicted to be the leading cause of death from cancer among women aged 20 to 59 years and the second leading cause of death for all women in 2016.[1] The median age for death from breast cancer is 68 years, with the age of 62 years for black women and 70 years for white women.[3]

The Cancer Intervention and Surveillance Modeling Network (CISNET) reported a decrease in the death rates from breast cancer from 1975 to 2000. The rate of death

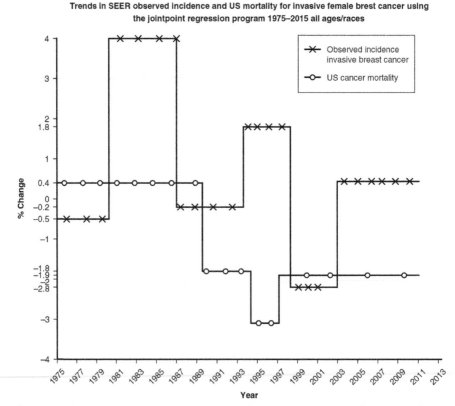

Fig. 1. Trends in the SEER program observed incidence and US mortality for invasive female breast cancer for all ages and races from 1975 through 2015.

from breast cancer adjusted for age to the 2000 population was 48.3 deaths per 100,000 women aged 30 to 79 years in 1975. By 1990 the rate was slightly increased to 49.7 per 100,000 but then it decreased to 38 per 100,000 by 2000, which was a decrease of 24% from 1990.[5] Another study documented a decrease in breast cancer deaths by 36% from 1989 to 2012.[3]

The annual percentage change in the mortalities from invasive breast cancer decreased by 1.3% from 1992 to 1995, decreased by 3.5% from 1995 to 1998, and decreased by 1.9% from 1998 to 2013.[4]

The trend for the incidence of female breast cancer had the greatest increase between 1980 and 1987; however, there has been minimal change since then. Meanwhile, the incidence of mortality from invasive breast cancer has continued to decline since 1975, most consistently since 1990. One report suggests that the incidence is more closely related to trends in factors that affect the cause, whereas mortality is affected by trends in treatment.[6] A question is whether the decreased mortality is largely caused by improved treatment,[7,8] mammographic screening,[9-14] or a combination of the two.[15]

RECOMMENDED SCREENING
Mammogram

Although there is no consensus on optimal strategies, target populations, or the harms and benefits,[16] screening mammography is the most commonly used method for the detection of breast cancer in women of average risk. Average risk is defined as the absence of a known susceptibility gene mutation (e.g BRCA1/BRC2), the absence of a history of previous breast cancer or ductal carcinoma in situ(DCIS), the absence of a family history of breast cancer, the absence of a history of lobular neoplasia or proliferative lesions on prior biopsy or chest irradiation.[14,17]

Screening mammography was associated with a decrease in the incidence of breast cancer by approximately 20% for women of all ages in a 2015 report.[14] However, some have expressed concern for overdiagnosis of breast cancer and risks/harms based on the timing and frequency of screening mammograms.[16,18-22]

The American College of Obstetricians and Gynecologists (ACOG), the National Comprehensive Cancer Network (NCCN), the American College of Radiology (ACR), the American Medical Association (AMA), the American College of Surgeons (ACS), and the National Cancer Institute (NCI) recommend annual screening mammography beginning at age 40 years.[9,23,24] The ACOG recommendation is level B, defined as recommendation based on limited or inconsistent scientific evidence.[23]

The US Preventive Services Task Force (USPSTF) recommends:

1. Against routine screening mammogram in women aged 40 to 49 years.
   - This recommendation is grade C, defined as "Recommends selective offering or providing to individual patients based on professional judgement and patient preferences (at least moderate certainty of small net benefit)."[25] The Affordable Care Act (ACA) leaves the discretion to payers regarding coverage for a grade C recommendation, whereas grades A and B are mandated to be covered with no cost sharing.
2. Biennial screening mammography is recommended for women aged 50–74 years as a grade B recommendation.
   - This recommendation is defined as a "high certainty that net benefit is moderate or moderate certainty that net benefit is moderate to substantial."[25]

3. There is no recommendation for screening after 74 years of age.
   - This recommendation is an I grade, defined as "Concludes that current evidence is insufficient to assess balance of benefits and harms of the service; evidence is lacking, of poor quality or conflicting and balance of benefits and harms cannot be determined."[25] As with the grade C recommendation, the ACA leaves the discretion to payers regarding coverage.[25,26]

The American Cancer Society recommends:

1. Regular screening beginning at age 45 years with annual mammograms until age 54 years as a strong recommendation.
   - This recommendation is defined as "most individuals should receive the recommended course of action..."
2. Women 55 years of age and older are recommended to begin biennial screening with the opportunity to continue annual screening as a qualified recommendation.
   - A qualified recommendation is defined as "Clinicians should acknowledge that different choices will be appropriate for different patients and that clinicians must help each patient arrive at a management decision consistent with his or her values and preferences..."
3. Women between the ages of 40 and 44 years should have the opportunity to have annual screening mammograms as a qualified recommendation.
4. There is no age established to stop mammograms but the recommendation is to continue as long as there is an overall life expectancy of at least 10 years and the overall health is good, as a qualified recommendation.[27]

Clinical Breast Examination, Breast Self-examination, Breast Self-examination Instruction, and Breast Self-awareness

Clinical breast examinations (CBEs) are recommended every 1 to 3 years from 20 to 39 years of age and annually beginning at age 40 years by ACOG (level C recommendation: Recommendation based primarily on consensus and expert opinion) and NCCN.[23] The ACS guidelines released in 2015 do not recommend CBE for breast cancer screening among average-risk women at any age as a qualified recommendation.[27-29] The USPSTF recommendation states that the current evidence is insufficient to assess the additional benefits and harms of clinical breast examination beyond screening mammography in women 40 years of age or older (I statement).[30]

The recommendations for breast self-examination, breast self-examination instruction, and breast self-awareness are inter-related and are considered together here. ACOG had recommended breast self-examination instruction for high-risk patients and the NCCN recommended it for all women. However, for these two groups there has been a movement away from this teaching toward breast self-awareness as a level C recommendation from ACOG.[23] The 2003 ACS guidelines did not include a recommendation for routine performance of, or instruction in, breast self-examination. There was no change in the 2015 guidelines.[27] The USPSTF 2009 guidelines recommend against clinicians teaching women how to perform breast self-examination as a grade D recommendation,[30] defined as moderate to high certainty of no net benefit or that harms outweigh benefits.[27] The USPSTF guidelines did not address self breast exam or self-awareness.

Risks and Benefits of Screening Mammogram, Breast Self-examination, Breast Self-examination Instruction, Clinical Breast Examination, and Breast Awareness Recommendations

The greatest variation in mammogram screening recommendations is for women 40 to 49 years old. One study concluded that, if biennial mammography screening started at age 40 instead of 50 years, for every 1000 women screened there would be a median of 1 more cancer deaths averted, but 576 more false-positive results, 67 more benign biopsies, and 2 additional overdiagnosed cases.[16] Another study concluded that 1 in every 3400 women in their 40s screened over 10 years would avoid breast cancer death compared with those not screened.[26] One report found more anxiety, distress, and breast cancer worry in varying numbers among women aged 40 to 49 years with false-positive mammography results. Another observational study found that of the women aged 40 to 49 years who experienced pain with mammogram, 11% to 46% declined future screening.[17] These data may have contributed to the recommendation of the USPSTF to individualize mammography screening recommendations for women aged 40 to 49 years with the same recommendation from the ACS but for women aged 40 to 44 years.

One report concluded that mammography screening could possibly identify a non-palpable mass measuring 1 mm to 1 cm during its preclinical phase, considered to be approximately 3 years before it becomes palpable.[31] It has also been reported that the time from when a cancer can be detected by screening until it becomes symptomatic (the sojourn time) varies with age and is the shortest for women aged 40 to 49 years.[23] Several studies have documented that breast tumors grow faster in younger, premenopausal women than in older menopausal and postmenopausal women.[31,32] When data from women screened annually were compared with biannual screening from age 40 to 85 years, the proportion of tumors that were stage IIB or higher and larger than 15 mm was greater for premenopausal than postmenopausal women. These data may have contributed to the ACS recommendation for annual screening mammograms for women 45 to 54 years old.[33,34]

Other data show that beginning annual mammograms at age 40 years results in the most life years gained[35–37] as well as decreased mortality.[14,15,36] A potential benefit is the identification of women with high-risk lesions, such as atypical ductal hyperplasia (ADH), atypical lobular hyperplasia, flat epithelial atypia, and lobular carcinoma in situ. These women may benefit from chemopreventive medication to decrease the risk of developing breast cancer, or screening MRI to detect occult cancer not detected by mammogram. A diagnosis at an earlier stage with a smaller tumor leads to less toxic and better tolerated treatments.[24] Tumors detected at an early stage that are confined to the breast are more likely to be treated successfully, with 98% 5-year survival rate.[23] One study reported that, among women 40 to 49 years old, those diagnosed with breast cancer had an earlier stage of breast cancer with smaller tumor size compared with women who did not have a screening mammogram.[24] These data may have contributed to the recommendation by ACOG, NCCN, ACR, AMA, and NCI to begin annual screening mammograms at age 40 years.

The other controversial group is women aged 74 years and older. One study assessed comorbidity along with screening to evaluate the potential benefits for this age group. For women with no comorbidity, the benefits of screening mammography extended through ages 76 to 78 years; for women with mild comorbidity (history of myocardial infarction [MI], acute MI, ulcer or rheumatologic disease) it was 74 to 76 years; for women with moderate comorbidity (the presence of vascular disease, cardiovascular disease, paralysis or diabetes) it was 72 to 74 years; and for women with severe comorbidity (the presence of acquired immunodeficiency syndrome, mild or severe liver disease, chronic obstructive pulmonary disease, chronic renal failure, dementia, or congestive heart failure) it was 66 to 68 years.[37,38] These recommendations are based on a meta-analysis that estimates that an average of 10.7 years was required before 1 death from breast cancer could be prevented per 1000 women screened.[39] However, healthy patients may choose to continue screening when the mortality benefit is small but also when less aggressive treatment is needed.[37,38]

In 2002, a large, prospective, randomized trial on breast self-examination was published. There were 26,000 textile workers in Shanghai who were either randomized to a group that was taught breast self-examination or a control group that did not receive the training. After a decade there was no difference in the stage at diagnosis or survival between the two groups. The investigators concluded that breast self-examination was not an effective screening tool.[40]

Some recent reports have concluded that there is no direct evidence of an association between CBE alone or in addition to mammography and breast cancer mortality.[41,42] However, in areas without the availability of screening mammography, some studies concluded that both CBE and breast self-examination may be the only screening available and therefore could be effective in reducing breast cancer mortality.[30,43,44]

Even though breast self-examination is no longer taught to women of average risk for breast cancer, breast self-awareness is recommended by some clinicians.[10,23] It has been estimated that more than 70% of breast cancers in women younger than 50 years and approximately 50% of breast cancers in women older than 50 years are detected by women themselves.[23] Two reports conclude that women should be encouraged to be aware of the normal appearance and feel of their breasts and be encouraged to promptly report any changes.[10,23]

RISK FACTORS FOR BREAST CANCER

Women at increased risk for breast cancer include women who are BRCA1/BRCA2 mutation carriers, women with a mother or sister with premenopausal breast cancer, women with greater than or equal to 20% lifetime risk for breast cancer based on risk assessment, women with histories of mantle radiation received between the ages of 10 and 30 years, and women who have biopsy-proven lobular neoplasia, ADH, DCIS, invasive breast cancer, or ovarian cancer regardless of age.[9]

Risk Tools

Mathematical models exist that stratify risk for breast cancer.[10]

- The Gail model was one of the earliest models created
  - It is available at www.cancer.gov/bcrisktool/
- The IBIS model includes more risk factors than other models
  - It is available at http://www.ems-trials.org/riskevaluator/

Web sites are available for risk assessment and information on genetic testing for breast cancer.

- The USPSTF site is www.uspreventiveservicestaskforce.org
- The Agency for Healthcare Research and Quality Web site is www.preventiveservices.ahrq.gov

Web sites provide several forms/questionnaires online to aid in family history collection of data to help determine the genetic risk for cancer[45]

- www.familyhistory.hhs.gov/
- www.cdc.gov/genomics/activities/famhx.htm
- www.nsgc.org/consumer/family tree/index.cfm

Genetics

ACOG recommends a genetic risk assessment for women with a greater than 20% to 25% chance of having an inherited predisposition to breast and ovarian cancer (level A recommendation: recommendation based on good scientific evidence).[46]

Hereditary breast and ovarian cancer syndrome includes a variety of inherited cancer-susceptibility syndromes. The hallmarks of this syndrome are multiple affected individuals in several generations, breast cancer diagnosed at an early age, and the presence of both breast cancer and ovarian cancer in a single individual. Strategies to decrease the risk of breast cancer in these women may include surveillance, chemoprevention, and surgery.[46] Recommended surveillance includes clinical breast examination semiannually as well as both annual mammography and annual breast MRI beginning at age 25 years or sooner based on the family history.[10]

Dense Breasts

Women with extremely dense breasts have a 4-fold increased risk for breast cancer. They also have an 18-fold increased risk of interval cancer, defined as cancer detected soon after a normal mammogram based on clinical symptoms. These interval cancers tend to be more aggressive and larger and have a worse prognosis than screen-detected cancers.[47]

Dense breast tissue on mammogram decreases the sensitivity of screening mammogram, especially if the cancer lacks calcifications.[48] However, there is no evidence to support additional testing in women who do not have additional risk factors. In 2015, an ACOG Committee Opinion stated that it "does not recommend routine use of alternative or adjunctive tests to screening mammography in women with dense breasts who are asymptomatic and have no additional risk factors."[49]

Factors Affecting the Relative Risk of Breast Cancer

There is an estimated increased relative risk for breast cancer of 1 to 1.5 in women who:

- Have never had a full-term pregnancy
- Are aged 30 years or older at first birth
- Are current users of hormonal contraception
- Had menarche at less than 12 years
- Have late menopause (after age 55 years)
- Are using estrogen and progestin long-term
- Are obese during postmenopause[23,50,51]

For women aged 40 to 49 years with a greater than 2 increased relative risk, some studies recommend screening mammograms before age 50 years.[22,50]

BENIGN BREAST DISORDERS
Palpable Breast Mass

The evaluation of a breast mass begins with a detailed history, assessment for breast cancer risk, and physical examination. Age-appropriate imaging can then be recommended. For women younger than 30 years, with a palpable mass, ultrasonography is the preferred initial modality. For women 30 years of age or older with a palpable mass, diagnostic mammography should be obtained with additional imaging with ultrasonography often required. Close clinical follow-up, biopsy, or both should be considered in the case of a discrete palpable mass with negative or discordant imaging results (ACOG level C recommendations).[52]

For women younger than 30 years, if the clinical suspicion for malignancy is low, the mass can be observed for 1 to 2 menstrual cycles with no imaging studies. If the mass resolves, no follow-up is needed but, if it persists, ultrasonography is the preferred initial testing.[52] One study documented a higher sensitivity for ultrasonography compared with mammogram (95.7% vs 60.9%) for women 30 to 39 years old.[51] If the ultrasonography detects a simple cyst, no further testing is necessary. However, if the mass is suspicious, if it is solid on ultrasonography, or if clinical suspicion is high, a mammogram is the next imaging study recommended.[51,52]

For women 30 years of age and older who have evaluation of a mass with a mammogram that shows a definitely benign mass and the clinical suspicion is low, no further testing is necessary.[51] For the remainder of these women, the next testing is ultrasonography[52] with subsequent individualization of care.

One study recommends that women from 30 to 39 years of age can have either an ultrasonography scan or a diagnostic mammogram for the initial evaluation of a palpable mass with the recommendation for diagnostic mammography as the initial testing at age 40 years.[51]

Nipple Discharge

Nipple discharge is the third most common complaint after palpable masses and pain for women presenting to a breast clinic. It is rarely the presenting symptom of cancer.[53] Benign discharge is multiductal and is more likely to be bilateral, milky, or green and only present when expressed. Bilateral milky discharge can occur during pregnancy and lactation and persist for up to 1 year postpartum or after the completion of breastfeeding. It can be caused by certain medications or from increased prolactin level or hypothyroidism.[52]

Discharge that is more suspicious is unilateral; from a single duct; spontaneous; persistent; and clear, serous, serosanguinous, or bloodstained.[53] If the discharge is considered to be pathologic, the first imaging study is a sonogram with the possible addition of a mammogram.[52,54,55] If both tests are negative, the management is individualized. Some patients may proceed to duct exploration and excision. Others may have additional imaging, such as a diagnostic ductography and MRI of the breast. The sensitivity of mammography in these patients was only 15%, whereas directed ultrasonography had a sensitivity of 56%.[55]

Papillary lesions are common among women aged 30 to 50 years and classically present with spontaneous nipple discharge. If the lesion is near the nipple it may manifest as a pathologic bloody discharge. Intraductal papillomas are benign and 50% are single lesions. However, there are atypical and malignant lesions with a chance of malignancy ranging from 3% to14%. Papillary carcinoma is more common in women older than 60 years.[53,54]

Duct ectasia is a benign condition that may cause bilateral viscous nipple discharge from multiple ducts. It is characterized by a dilatation of the mammary ducts and usually is managed conservatively.[54]

Breast Pain

Breast pain (mastalgia) is experienced by as many as 10% to 30% of women.[56] It is classified as:

1. Cyclic, which has a clear relationship to the menstrual cycle.
2. Noncyclic, which can be constant or intermittent and is not associated with the menstrual cycle. Most of these women are perimenopausal or postmenopausal.

3. Extramammary, which arises from the chest wall or other sources, but is considered to be breast pain. Most likely it is secondary to costochondritis and other syndromes, including fibromyalgia, cervical radiculopathy, herpes zoster, angina, and gastroesophageal reflux disease.[52,57]

Cyclic mastalgia can interfere with sleep, physical activity, work or school, social functioning, and sexual activity. Studies including histologic, hormonal, fluid, nutritional, and psychological causes have not shown conclusive results.[57]

Likewise, noncyclic mastalgia has an unknown cause and can affect the quality of life. It tends to be unilateral and localized within a quadrant of the breast. It is thought to be more likely to have an anatomic rather than hormonal cause.[57]

A common reason for evaluation of breast pain is the fear of cancer. If the only symptom is breast pain, and there are no risk factors, the risk of cancer is low. A mammogram and/or sonogram should be ordered based on abnormalities noted on physical examination.[54] Women with normal findings on clinical examination and a normal mammographic evaluation for breast pain had an estimated risk of 0.5% for occult cancer.[57]

Most women responded to reassurance after normal findings; however, some required additional intervention. Nonpharmacologic measures that were beneficial for some patients included improved mechanical support with counseling on the use and selection of a properly fitting brassiere, exercise, relaxation training, and caffeine restriction or elimination.[57] Evening primrose oil was beneficial for some women but studies showed conflicting results. Women with severe breast pain causing a negative impact on their quality of life were shown in some studies to derive benefit from medications such as danazol or tamoxifen. Use of these medications is not frequent because of the concern for adverse side effects.[57]

Skin Changes

The most common skin disorders of breasts evaluated in a dermatology clinic were melanocytic or nonmelanocytic proliferation (nevi and seborrheic keratosis), cysts, or reexcision of these lesions. They accounted for 76% of the biopsies. Approximately 4% of the biopsies showed metastatic carcinoma, almost all from primary breast cancer.

Most skin disorders of the breast are similar to those found on the abdomen, which is another sun-protected truncal area.[58] These diagnoses include psoriasis, eczema, and contact dermatitis. Skin changes such as peau d'orange (skin edema) and erythema may indicate breast cancer.[52]

The nipple-areolar area has a different set of potential diagnoses. In one study, 40% of the biopsies from the nipple and 60% from the areola represented inflammatory dermatoses, with most being spongiotic dermatitis or chronic dermatitis. Bilateral involvement of the nipple-areolar area favors a benign process.

The dermatitislike Paget disease is most commonly unilateral. It can appear as typical eczema or nipple erosion or ulceration. Most women with Paget disease have a clinical abnormality of the nipple. Underlying DCIS is detected in more than 90% of patients with Paget disease. It is multifocal in approximately 50% of the cases and does not necessarily occur near or contiguous with the nipple-areolar area.[58] Nipple eczema is a characteristic manifestation of atopic dermatitis. Friction against clothing may cause irritant dermatitis, referred to as jogger's nipples. Basal cell carcinoma and squamous cell carcinoma rarely involve the nipple.[58]

Inflammatory Breast Disorders

Lactational mastitis is the most common form of mastitis, occurring in 1% to 24% of breastfeeding women.[53] Treatment includes antibiotics and encouragement of milk flow from the engorged area. Approximately 5% to 11% of these women develop an abscess, which can be confirmed with ultrasonography and managed with aspiration of the fluid or incision and drainage. If inflammation does not resolve with treatment, imaging studies, including sonogram and/or mammogram, may be indicated to assess for associated masses or evidence of malignancy.[54]

Nonlactational infections are classified according to location, either central (periareolar) or peripheral. These infections include periductal mastitis; granulomatous lobular mastitis; and skin-associated infections, including infected epidermal cysts and cellulitis of the breast. Tobacco smoking is significantly associated with 90% of patients who develop periductal mastitis. Nipple piercing is associated with a 10% to 20% risk. Other risk factors include diabetes, black race, and obesity.[53] These infections and abscesses are treated similarly to lactating infections and abscesses. Recurrent infections are more common than among lactating abscesses and may require surgery. However, as with lactational infections, if the inflammation does not resolve with treatment, imaging studies may be indicted to evaluate for evidence of malignancy.[54]

Inflammatory breast cancer is the most aggressive presentation of breast cancer. The incidence ranges from 1% to 5% of breast cancers. In 2010 an international panel was convened to standardize the diagnosis and treatment of this cancer. Minimal criteria for the diagnosis include:

1. A history of rapid onset of breast erythema, edema and/or peau d'orange, and/or warm breast, with or without an underlying palpable mass
2. Clinical examination revealing erythema occupying at least one-third of the breast
3. Duration of history of no more than 6 months
4. Pathologic confirmation of invasive carcinoma from a core biopsy of the breast[59]

ADOLESCENTS

Adolescent women commonly have concerns about their breasts, ranging from nipple discharge to pain to appearance.[54] When adolescents present for medical examination, the first step is often education and reassurance regarding normal variation in anatomy, growth, and development. They should also be screened for body dysmorphic disorder as recommended in an ACOG Committee Opinion.[60]

Palpable Breast Mass

For adolescents with a palpable solid breast mass, sonography is the recommended testing.[54] The most common solid breast lesion in adolescents is fibroadenoma, comprising 86.4% of breast masses in one study involving adolescents.[61] The natural history of fibroadenomas is slow growth and eventual regression. It has been estimated that 16% to 37% resolve within 1 to 3 years and 30% reduce in size within 5 years.[61]

Primary malignant pediatric breast lesions are rare, with a prevalence reported as less than 0.1%. The age-related rate for sarcomatous malignant pediatric breast tumors was reported as 0.06 per 100,000 adolescents with phyllodes tumors as the most common type. The sonographic findings of benign and malignant phyllodes tumors overlap. Tissue sampling is needed to diagnose the type.

Because of the low risk of malignancy in adolescents and the possibility of a reduction in the size of fibroadenomas over a 2-year period, some clinicians have recommended sonographic monitoring of asymptomatic fibroadenomas measuring less than 5 cm and using the combined criteria of size and volume change per month as an alternative to tissue sampling. It has been recommended to continue 6-month sonographic testing until the resolution of the mass or age 29 years.[61]

Breast Asymmetry

During puberty it is common to have asymmetric breast growth. If no mass is palpable, one study advises that patients and their parents can be counseled that asymmetry often becomes less noticeable with age.[54]

Juvenile Hypertrophy of the Breasts

Juvenile hypertrophy is extreme macromastia with pathologic overgrowth of both breasts with the onset of menarche. Each breast may weigh as much as 15 to 20 kg (30–50 pounds). Surgical management is often considered in older teens or young adults.[54]

Breast Reduction Surgery

Breast reduction surgery in adolescents with large breasts can relieve back, neck, and shoulder pain. Recommendations for timing of the surgery include postponing surgery until breast maturity is reached, until there is stability in the cup size over 6 months, and waiting until the age of 18 years. Before surgery it is recommended to assess the adolescent's emotional, physiologic, and physical maturity.[60]

Breast Augmentation

Breast augmentation in adolescents may be performed for reconstruction of congenital deformities or severe asymmetry or as an elective procedure to augment small breast size or mild asymmetry. The American Society of Plastic Surgeons recommends that women considering breast augmentation should:

1. Be at least 18 years of age before undergoing the surgery
2. Have the necessary physical and emotional maturity to ensure the most positive outcome
3. Have a realistic understanding of the potential results, as well as the possible need for additional surgery[60]

REFERENCES

1. Siegel RL, Miller KD, Jemal A. Cancer statistics, 2016. CA Cancer J Clin 2016;66: 7–30.
2. Siegel RL, Miller KD, Jemal A. Cancer statistics, 2015. CA Cancer J Clin 2015;65: 5–29.
3. DeSantis CE, Fedewa SA, Sauer AG, et al. Breast cancer statistics, 2015. convergence of incidence rates between black and white women. CA Cancer J Clin 2016;66:31–42.
4. Howlader N, Noone AM, Krapcho M, et al. SEER cancer statistics review 1975-2013. National Cancer Institute; 2015.
5. Berry DA, Cronin KA, Plevritis SK, et al. Effect of screening and adjuvant therapy on mortality from breast cancer. N Engl J Med 2005;353:1784–92.
6. Holford TR, Cronin KA, Mariotto AB, et al. Changing patterns in breast cancer incidence trends. J Natl Cancer Inst Monogr 2006;36:19–25.

7. Bleyer A, Welch HG. Effect of three decades of screening mammography on breast-cancer incidence. N Engl J Med 2012;367:1998–2005.

8. Bleyer A, Baines C, Miller AB. Impact of screening mammography on breast cancer mortality. Int J Control 2016;138(8):2003–12.

9. Lee CH, Dershaw D, Kopans D, et al. Breast cancer screening with imaging: recommendations from the society of breast imaging and the ACR on the use of mammography, breast MRI, breast ultrasound and other technologies for the detection of clinically occult breast cancer. J Am Coll Radiol 2010;7:18–27.

10. Euhus D, DiCarlo PA, Khouri NF. Breast cancer screening. Surg Clin NA 2015; 95(5):991–1011.

11. Chetlen A, Mack J, Chan T. Breast cancer screening controversies: who, when, why and how? Clin Imaging 2015;40(2):279–82.

12. Swain M, Jeudy M, Pearlman MD. Controversies in screening mammography. Clin Ob Gyn 2016;59(2):351–61.

13. American College of Obstetricians and Gynecologists. Practice advisory: breast cancer screening. 2016. Available at: http://www.acog.org. Accessed May 19, 2016.

14. Myers ER, Moorman P, Gierisch JM, et al. Benefits and harms of breast cancer screening. a systematic review. JAMA 2015;314(15):1615–34.

15. Malmgren JA, Parikh J, Atwood MK, et al. Impact of mammography detection on the course of breast cancer in women aged 40-49. Radiology 2012;262(3): 797–806.

16. Mandelblatt JS, Stout NK, Schechter CB, et al. Collaborative modeling of the benefits and harms associated with different US breast cancer screening strategies. Ann Intern Med 2016;164(4):215–25.

17. Nelson HD, Pappas M, Cantor A, et al. Harms of breast cancer screening: systematic review to update the 2009 US preventive services task force recommendation. Ann Intern Med 2016;164(4):256–67.

18. Pace LE, Keating NL. A systematic assessment of benefits and risks to guide breast cancer screening decisions. JAMA 2014;311(13):1327–35.

19. Keen JD, Jorgensen KJ. Four principles to consider before advising women on screening mammography. J Womens Health (Larchmt) 2015;24(11):867–74.

20. Crosswell JM, Ransohoff DF, Kramer BS. Principles of cancer screening: lessons from history and study design issues. Semin Oncol 2010;37(3):202–15.

21. Harding C, Pompei F, Burmistov D, et al. Breast cancer screening, incidence and mortality across US. Counties JAMA Intern Med 2015;175(9):1483–9.

22. Siu AL. Screening for breast cancer: US preventive services task force recommendation statement. Ann Intern Med 2016;164(4):279–96.

23. American College of Obstetricians and Gynecologists. Practice bulletin no. 122: breast cancer screening. Obstet Gynecol 2011;118:372–82.

24. Plecha D, Salem N, Kremer M, et al. Journal club: neglecting to screen women between 40 and 49 years old with mammography: what is the impact on treatment morbidity and potential risk reduction? Am J Dermatopathol 2014;202: 282–8.

25. Siu AL, Bibbins-Domingo K, Grossman D. Evidence-based clinical prevention in the era of the patient protection and affordable care act. The role of the US preventive services task force. JAMA 2015;314(19):2012–22.

26. Lin KW, Gostin LO. A public health framework for screening mammography. Evidence-based vs politically mandated care. JAMA 2016;315(10):977–8.

27. Oeffinger KC, Fontham ETH, Etsioni R, et al. Breast cancer screening for women at average risk. 2015 guidelines update from the American Cancer Society. JAMA 2015;314(15):1599–614.
28. Bredemeyer M. ACS releases guideline on breast cancer screening. Am Fam Physician 2016;93(8):711–2.
29. Keating NL, Pace LE. New guidelines for breast cancer screening in US Women. JAMA 2015;314(15):1569–71.
30. US Preventive Services Task Force. Screening for breast cancer: US Preventive Services Task Force recommendation statement. Ann Intern Med 2009;151(10): 716–26.
31. Macdonald I. The natural history of mammary carcinoma. Am J Surg 1966;111: 435–42.
32. White E, Miglioretti DL, Yankaskas BC, et al. Biennial versus annual mammography and the risk of late-stage breast cancer. J Natl Cancer Inst 2004;96: 1832–9.
33. Fenichel M. American Cancer Society changes breast cancer screening guidelines to reflect analysis of benefits and harms. J Natl Cancer Inst 2016;108(2). pii: djw022.
34. Hubbard RA, Kerlikowske K, Flowers CI, et al. Cumulative probability of false positive recall or biopsy recommendation after 10 years of screening mammography. Ann Intern Med 2011;155:481–92.
35. Keating NL, Pace LE. Screening mammography and age recommendations. JAMA 2016;315(13):1403–4.
36. Helvie MA. USPSTF erroneously understated life-years-gained benefit of mammographic screening of women in their 40's. Radiology 2011;258(3):958–9.
37. Lansdorp-Vogelaar I, Gulati R, Mariotto AB, et al. Personalizing age of cancer screening cessation based on comorbid conditions: model estimates of harms and benefits. Ann Intern Med 2014;161:104–12.
38. Braithwaite D, Walter LC, Izano M, et al. Benefits and harms of screening mammography by comorbidity and age: a qualitative synthesis of observational studies and decision analyses. J Gen Intern Med 2016;31(5):561–72.
39. Lee SJ, Boscardin WJ, Stijacic-Cenzer I, et al. Time lag to benefit after screening for breast and colorectal cancer: meta- analysis of survival data from the United States, Sweden, United Kingdom and Denmark. BMJ 2012;345:e8441–9.
40. Mark K, Temkin SM, Terplan M. Breast self-awareness. The evidence behind the euphemism. Obstet Gynecol 2014;123:734–6.
41. Elmore JG, Reisch LM, Barton MB, et al. Efficacy of breast cancer screening in the community according to risk level. J Natl Cancer Inst 2005;97:1035–43.
42. Oestreicher N, Lehman CD, Seger DJ, et al. The incremental contribution of clinical breast examination to invasive cancer detection in a mammography screening program. AJR Am J Roentgenol 2005;184:428–32.
43. Anderson BO, Bevers TB, Carlson RW. Clinical breast examination and breast cancer screening guideline. JAMA 2016;315(13):1403–4.
44. Hassan LM, Mahmoud N, Miller AB, et al. Evaluation of effect of self-examination and physical examination on breast cancer. The Breast 2015;24:487–90.
45. Rodabaugh K, Brewer MA, Chalas E, et al. Focus on female cancers: hereditary breast and ovarian cancer. American College of Obstetricians and Gynecologists, District II/NY. 2008. p. 1–42. Available at: www.acogny.org.
46. The American College of Obstetricians and Gynecologists. Practice bulletin no. 103: hereditary breast and ovarian cancer syndrome. Obstet Gynecol 2009; 113:957–66.

47. Berg WA. Supplemental breast cancer screening in women with dense breasts should be offered with simultaneous collection of outcomes data. Ann Intern Med 2016;164(4):299–300.

48. Green VL. Mammographic breast density and breast cancer risk: implications of breast density legislation for health care practitioners. Clin Obstet Gynecol 2016; 59(2):419–38.

49. The American College of Obstetricians and Gynecologists. Management of women with dense breasts diagnosed by mammography. Committee Opinion no. 625. Obstet Gynecol 2015;125:750–1.

50. Nelson HD, Zakher B, Cantor A, et al. Risk factors for breast cancer for women aged 40-49 years: a systematic review and meta-analysis. Ann Intern Med 2012;156(9):635–48.

51. Harvey JA, Mahoney MC, Newell MS, et al. ACR appropriateness criteria palpable breast masses. J Am Coll Radiol 2013;10:742–9.

52. The American College of Obstetricians and Gynecologists. Diagnosis and management of benign breast disorders. Practice bulletin no. 164. Obstet Gynecol 2016;127:e141–56.

53. Amin AL, Purdy AC, Mattingly JD, et al. Benign breast disease. Surg Clin North Am 2013;93:299–308.

54. Onstad M, Stuckey A. Benign breast disorders. Obstet Gynecol Clin North Am 2013;40:459–73.

55. Bahl M, Baker JA, Greenup RA, et al. Diagnostic value of ultrasound in female patients with nipple discharge. AJR Am J Roentgenology 2015;205:203–8.

56. Khan SA, Apkarian AV. Mastalgia and breast cancer: a protective association? Cancer Detect Prev 2002;26:192–6.

57. Smith RL, Pruthi S, Fitzpatrick LA. Evaluation and management of breast pain. Mayo Clinic Proc 2004;79(3):353–72.

58. Peters MS, Lehman JS, Comfere NI. Dermatology of the female breast. Am J Dermatopathol 2013;35(3):289–307.

59. Dawood S, Merajver SD, Viens P, et al. International expert panel on inflammatory breast cancer: consensus statement for standardized diagnosis and treatment. Ann Oncol 2011;22:515–23.

60. American College of Obstetricians and Gynecology. Breast and labial surgery in adolescents. Committee Opinion no 662. Obstet Gynecol 2016;127:e138–40.

61. Jawahar A, Vade A, Ward K, et al. Biopsy versus conservative management of sonographically benign-appearing solid breast masses in adolescents. J Ultrasound Med 2015;34:617–25.

Recognizing and Managing Common Urogynecologic Disorders

Denise M. Elser, MD

KEYWORDS

- Urogynecologic disorders • Urinary incontinence • Pelvic organ prolapse
- Management • Treatment • Surgery

KEY POINTS

- Many women experience urogynecologic or pelvic floor disorders, especially urinary incontinence and pelvic organ prolapse.
- The obstetrician/gynecologist is often the first health care professional who will have an opportunity to listen, and then evaluate and treat these disorders.
- A wide variety of treatments are available to treat incontinence, including pelvic floor muscle training, behavioral therapies, oral medications, neuromodulation, intradetrusor medications, and surgery.
- When approaching the woman with symptomatic prolapse, familiarity with pessaries and various surgical procedures will aid in appropriately counseling the patient.
- Referral to a pelvic floor physical therapist or to a female pelvic medicine and reconstructive surgeon should be considered. Increasing attention to data on cost-effectiveness is a necessity.

INTRODUCTION

For most women in the United States, the obstetrician/gynecologist (OB/GYN) is the one health care professional with whom they would ever dream of sharing their concerns related to urinary incontinence (UI) or pelvic organ prolapse (POP). For many women, incontinence or prolapse may be the issue that drives them back into the care of a physician after several years of feeling healthy and without perceived need of a medical professional.

The most common pelvic floor disorders addressed by the OB/GYN are UI and POP. Prevalence of incontinence is estimated at up to 55% of older women and 12% to 42% for younger and middle-aged women.[1] Although men also suffer from UI, women experience the condition disproportionately at up to 4.5 times higher rates. Prolapse is also highly prevalent, especially after menopause. Analysis of participants

Women's Health Institute of Illinois, 5851 West 95th Street, Suite 300, Oak Lawn, IL 60453, USA
E-mail address: delser@whii.org

Obstet Gynecol Clin N Am 44 (2017) 271–284
http://dx.doi.org/10.1016/j.ogc.2017.02.011
0889-8545/17/© 2017 Elsevier Inc. All rights reserved.

obgyn.theclinics.com

in the Women's Health Initiative Study found that at a mean age of 68.7 years, the baseline rate of stage 2 or higher prolapse was 70%.[2]

URINARY INCONTINENCE
Types of Urinary Incontinence

Generally, UI is categorized as stress, urge, or mixed incontinence. Less common causes are due to fistula, overflow, or ectopic ureter. We can refer to type of incontinence by symptoms: stress UI in which a woman complains of leakage with physical stress on the bladder, such as coughing, sneezing, jumping or lifting; urge incontinence, which is described as a strong urge to urinate with leakage before becoming fully seated on the toilet; or mixed incontinence for women with both stress UI and urge incontinence complaints. In the most recent International Urogynecology Association/International Continence Society consensus document on terminology, several other categories of incontinence symptoms have been awarded official terminology[3] (**Table 1**). The actual conditions may be referred to as urodynamics stress incontinence, in which cases that incontinence with cough or a Valsalva maneuver has been diagnosed by urodynamics testing; detrusor overactivity for cases in which uninhibited detrusor contractions have been identified during bladder filling; or urodynamic mixed incontinence, which refers to cases when both conditions are diagnosed by urodynamics.

Evaluation of Urinary Incontinence

Initially, patient history is used to determine if symptoms are stress, urge, or mixed. If mixed, it is pertinent to notate which component occurs more frequently or is more bothersome to the patient.

Assessment of the severity of UI may simply involve asking the patient how often she leaks and whether she leaks a small or large volume with each episode. Use of pads, the number of pads used, and the type of pad required provide a rough estimate

Table 1 Categories of urinary incontinence symptoms	
Term	**Definition**
Urinary incontinence	The involuntary loss of urine
Stress urinary incontinence	Urine leakage that occurs with physical stress such as laugh, cough, sneeze, lifting, etc
Urgency incontinence	Leakage that occurs with preceding urge to void
Postural incontinence	Urinary leakage that occurs with a change in position (such as sitting to standing)
Nocturnal enuresis	Urine leakage occurs during sleep
Mixed urinary incontinence	Leakage that occurs with physical stress and also with preceding urge to void
Continuous incontinence	Leakage occurs continuously
Insensible incontinence	Occurs without awareness of when or how leakage occurred
Coital incontinence	Complaint of loss of urine with sexual intercourse (penetration or orgasm)

Adapted from Haylen BT, De Ridder D, Freeman RM, et al. An International Urogynecological Association (IUGA)/International Continence Society (ICS) joint report on the terminology for female pelvic floor dysfunction. Neurourol Urodyn 2010;29(1):5; with permission.

of the amount of leakage. In general, increasing severity of incontinence will be found as a woman evolves from no pad, to panty liner, to menstrual pads, to incontinence pads to adult diapers. These products become increasingly bulky and more expensive along the spectrum; thus, when a woman spends the additional money, she is usually in need of additional protection from a greater volume or frequency of wetness. The basic difference between menstrual pads and incontinence pads is that the latter consist of beads made to absorb the less viscous urine, causing the beads to swell into a gel solid, much like an infant's diaper.

Voiding diaries are a low-tech method to determine the frequency of incontinence. A simple voiding diary may be logged for 3 to 7 days and consists of having the patient track when she urinates, and when she leaks with a notation as to what was happening when she leaked, such as "coughing," "Zumba class," or "urge." More detailed is the frequency–volume chart (**Table 2**). On the frequency–volume chart, the patient logs liquids consumed with amount, time of voiding with volume, any incontinence episodes and if and when pads are changed. Because the frequency–volume chart is quite cumbersome, usually this record is requested for 1 to 3 days. Providing the patient with a "Texas hat" or a urine hat facilitates measuring voided urine. Pad testing is a research tool and not clinically useful for the OB/GYN physician.

In the office evaluation, pelvic examination will note urogenital atrophy, presence of prolapse, tenderness, size of uterus, and assessment of pelvic floor muscles. Pelvic floor strength is assessed on a scale of 0 to 4, referred to as the Oxford Scale for grading pelvic floor muscle strength, with 0 representing no ability to squeeze and 4 representing a strong squeeze and elevation of perineum (**Table 3**).[4,5] During bimanual examination, the patient is asked to squeeze her pelvic muscles. Phrases such as "practice your Kegel," "imagine you are in public and have a need to pass gas—try to hold it in" are helpful in getting women to understand which muscles to use. Despite strong verbal cues, however, the majority of women with complaints of UI or POP have poor ability to contract their pelvic muscles. Our group assessed 325 women presenting for initial visit to a urogynecology clinic.[6] About three-quarters had heard of Kegel exercises, but only 40% had ever previously been instructed to perform them. Of those, the majority had received only verbal instructions. Fewer than one-quarter of women could contract with Oxford scale 3 or higher. Hypertonicity and/or tenderness of pelvic muscles should be assessed, but there is not an accepted scale to score these findings. The cough stress test—simply having a woman cough forcibly while

Table 2
Frequency/volume chart example

1—Time	2—Intake	3—Urination	4—Leaks	5—Pads
0500 AM				
0600 AM	6 oz OJ	400 mL		Incontinence pad
0700 AM				
0800 AM			✓ cough	
0900 AM	8 oz coffee			
1000 AM		200 mL		
1100 AM			✓✓✓ urge	+ pad

On the chart, patients record the following at the corresponding hour (column 1); column 2—what you drink, when and how much; column 3—urination with amounts; column 4—any incontinence episodes and any activity associated. Use 1 checkmark for a small amount of leakage up to 4 checkmarks for a large amount of leakage; column 5—if you changed your pad and which type.

Table 3
Oxford scale for grading pelvic floor muscle strength

Grade	Characteristics
0	No discernible contraction
1	Barely palpable, flickering contraction, not visible on inspection of the perineum
2	Weak, distinctly palpable contraction, felt as slight pressure on the examining finger
3	Moderate muscle strength, distinct pressure on the examining finger, and palpable upward and forward movement, visible on the perineal surface
4	Good muscle strength, elevation possible against slight resistance, circular pressure can be felt around the examining finger. During simultaneous examination by the index and middle finger these are pressed against each other
5	Very strong muscle strength, contraction possible against vigorous resistance, with suction-type effect on the examining finger

Data from Brink CA, Wells TJ, Sampselle CM, et al. A digital test for pelvic muscle strength in women with urinary incontinence. Nurs Res 1994;43(6):352–6; and Laycock J, Jerwood D. Development of the Bradford perineometer. Physiotherapy 1994;80:139–42.

examining the urethral meatus for evidence of leakage—is a critical part of the examination. Considering that most women experience UI with a somewhat full bladder in an upright position and gynecologist examinations typically occur in the dorsolithotomy position after a woman has voided, it may be necessary to have the patient stand and cough to demonstrate stress UI. If the supine empty cough stress test is positive, however, this is suspicious for severe UI known as intrinsic sphincteric deficiency. In fact, the negative supine cough stress test has a 70% sensitivity for predicting intrinsic sphincteric deficiency and 98% predictive value for diagnosing stress UI.[7]

The remainder of the basic assessment involves screening for urinary tract infection with urinalysis, measuring post void residual via ultrasound, or in-and-out catheterization. Using a catheterized measurement is more accurate than an ultrasound measurement. The amount of "residual" urine is affected by the duration of time that passes between a void and the measurement. Normal post void residual in women remains unclear, but is widely accepted that an upper limit of 100 mL measured within 10 minutes of a void is normal.[8] An isolated elevated post void residual measurement is not cause for alarm. Persistently elevated residuals deserve further evaluation.

Urodynamics testing involves flowmetry or an assessment of voiding function and then cystometry or study of bladder filling. Using a pressure tip catheter via the urethra, the bladder is filled with saline while bladder and or urethral pressures are measured. The intraabdominal pressure is estimated via a vaginal or rectal pressure catheter. Testing measures bladder sensation (first sensation, urge to void, strong desire, and pain), examines for evidence of uninhibited detrusor contractions during bladder filling (detrusor overactivity) and studies urethral function during stress episodes such as standing, coughing and bearing down. A pressure–flow study, in which a woman voids on a commode with the bladder and vaginal catheters in place measures if a woman's voiding mechanism uses urethral relaxation, detrusor contraction, or use of Valsalva or some combination of the above. The pressure–flow study may provide helpful information to predict the probability of voiding dysfunction after incontinence surgery (**Figs. 1** and **2**).

Not all women require urodynamics testing before the initiation of treatment. Urodynamics are indicated if the basic evaluation cannot guide treatment, after failed conservative therapy, and before surgery for stress incontinence if stress UI has not been demonstrated during examination, for women older than age 60, and those who

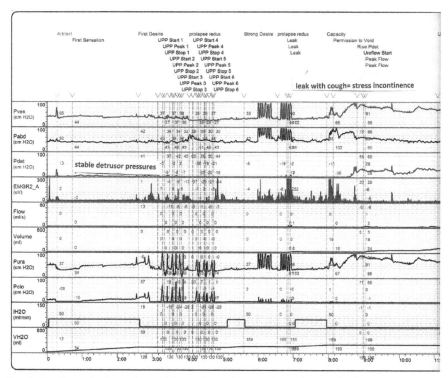

Fig. 1. Urodynamics in patient with urodynamic stress incontinence (USI).

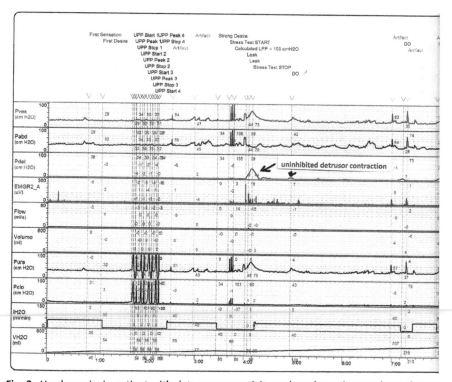

Fig. 2. Urodynamics in patient with detrusor overactivity and urodynamic stress incontinence.

have undergone prior incontinence procedures. Urodynamics may also be performed before prolapse repair. In a 2012, the American Urogynecologic Society issued a position statement stating that urodynamics are not necessary if a woman has uncomplicated stress dominant incontinence, a positive office stress test, normal postvoid residual, and a normal urinalysis.[9] The statement did not address women with previous surgery, concomitant prolapse, urge predominant incontinence, or neurologic disease.

Cystoscopy is not indicated in the routine evaluation of UI.[10] Indications for cystoscopy are hematuria (microscopic or gross), intractable or rapid onset urge incontinence, recurrent urinary tract infection, if fistula or urethral diverticulum are suspected, or if the patient has had prior surgery with permanent suture, such as a Burch procedure, or prior pelvic mesh for prolapse or sling.

Conservative Management of Urinary Incontinence

When a women presents with UI, treatment can be initiated before a specific diagnosis is determined. Once we have ruled out urinary tract infection, pelvic mass, significant POP, and elevated residual, then treatment should be offered and may be based on the predominant symptom, either stress or urge. All women presenting for treatment of UI should be presented with options for conservative therapy as well as more invasive options. Conservative therapy options include pelvic muscle exercises, alone or with pelvic floor physical therapy, behavioral therapies, pessaries, and medication.

Behavioral therapies run a wide gamut of areas that can impact bladder function. These begin with avoiding or decreasing caffeine intake, assessing excess fluid intake,[11] losing weight if the body mass index is greater than 30 kg/m^2,[12] and control of constipation if present, because constipation can negatively impact bladder function, especially urge incontinence. Most research supporting treating constipation to improve urgency and urge incontinence has been performed in children and the elderly, but this concept applies to women of all ages.[13,14] Diabetes is a risk factor for UI, especially type 2 diabetes mellitus. Weight loss has been shown to improve bladder control in diabetics.[15,16] Further, it is very difficult to treat urgency and urge incontinence if significant glycosuria is present. As alluded to, performing Kegel exercises at home with only verbal instruction may be poorly effective because the majority of women with urinary complaints cannot contract their pelvic muscles well. A Cochrane review concluded that pelvic floor muscle training should be offered as a first-line therapy for all women with stress, urge, or mixed UI.[17] Treatment of urge incontinence may focus on downtraining hypertonic muscles and release of trigger points, rather than straight muscle strengthening, and is thus another reason that home exercise alone may not be beneficial. Vaginal pessaries intended for prolapse control, or those specifically designed to control incontinence, can be offered with little risk to the patient. However, in this evolving atmosphere of cost-effective medicine, we need to understand that frequent visits for comfort, a poorly fitting pessary, discharge or spotting, and lack of efficacy can cause the pessary to be fairly expensive. One study found that at 1 year, both pessaries and pelvic floor muscle training were found to be less cost effective than midurethral sling for the initial treatment of stress UI.[18]

Pharmacologic therapy can be offered to women with urge or mixed symptoms of UI. Increasingly, third-party payors require a trial of an anticholinergic medication before authorization of more invasive procedures. Common muscarinic side effects are dry eyes, dry mouth, or constipation. Of the anticholinergics available to treat overactive bladder, trospium is the only one that has been demonstrated not to cross the blood-brain barrier.[19] It is important to be aware of polypharmacy, especially in the elderly, and to be aware of the combined anticholinergic burden and potential for effect on mentation in any given patient. Anticholinergic medications should not be prescribed to patients with narrow-angle glaucoma and used with caution in those with gastroesophageal reflux and urinary retention.

In addition to the anticholinergics, the only other medication approved by the US Food and Drug Administration to treat overactive bladder is mirabegron, a beta 3 adrenergic agonistic.[20] Because this medication can increase blood pressure and result in headaches, a blood pressure check within 1 to 2 weeks of initiating mirabegron is recommended.

Dual therapy, referring to 2 different prescription medications for overactive bladder, may be prescribed if symptoms are managed suboptimally by 1 drug, if the medications are of different categories and well-tolerated by the patient. However, patients are poorly compliant with long-term prescriptions for 1 overactive bladder drug, let alone 2.

Procedures in Urinary Incontinence—Overactive Bladder

The joint guidelines[21] published in 2014 by the American Urologic Association (AUA) and the Society of Urodynamics and Female Urology recommend allowing 8 to 12 weeks for behavioral therapy and 4 to 8 weeks for pharmacologic therapies. These guidelines recommend education, behavioral therapy, and then pharmacologic treatment. Fourth-line treatment for overactive bladder include neuromodulation or intravesical injection of onabotulinumtoxinA (Botox). There are currently 2 widely available categories of neuromodulation: posterior tibial nerve stimulation, known as brand name, Urgent PC, or implantable sacral neuromodulator, known as sacral nerve stimulation or by the brand name, Interstim.

Posterior tibial nerve stimulation is performed in the office setting with recommended 12 weekly 30-minute stimulation procedures. The technique involves the placement of a 34-gauge (acupuncture) needles just under the skin 4 to 5 cm cephalad to the medial malleolus. Stimulation via a small handheld device is applied. Proper placement is confirmed when movement of the toes, and in particular flexion of the big toe, occurs. The current is increased based on patient tolerability and is set just under the pain threshold.[22]

Posterior tibial nerve stimulation was compared with sham stimulation in a blinded study of 220 patient with overactive bladder symptoms.[23] Analysis found that 54.5% experienced moderate or marked improvement in overactive bladder compared with 20.9% in the sham group. No serious adverse events have been reported in the literature to date. The most common complaint is mild pain at the needle insertion site.

OnabotulinumtoxinA is indicated for the treatment of refractory idiopathic overactive bladder or neuropathic overactive bladder. The term neuropathic overactive bladder indicates that there is a known brain, spinal cord, or nerve condition causing detrusor overactivity. The remainder of this discussion refers to idiopathic overactive bladder only.

A systematic review of the use of onabotulinumtoxinA in treating refractory idiopathic overactive bladder in men and women examined the literature published between 1985 and 2009.[24] Pooled data determined that onabotulinumtoxinA patients experienced about 4 fewer incontinence episodes per day. Risks include elevated post void residuals and symptomatic urinary retention. Lower doses of onabotulinumtoxinA of 100 to 150 units are associated with lower risk of retention but higher doses seem to have longer lasting benefits. Patients receiving repeated doses of onabotulinumtoxinA do not become refractory to the drug with subsequent injections.

Sacral nerve stimulation is a surgically implanted stimulator, physically similar to a cardiac pacemaker. The small stimulator is placed subdermally in the buttocks region attached to a unilateral lead also placed subcutaneously that stimulates the S3 nerve root. Indications are overactive bladder, urinary retention, fecal incontinence, and constipation.

In 1 randomized, controlled trial, 147 patients were assigned to standard medical therapy or sacral nerve stimulation and evaluated for efficacy at 6 months.[25] An intention-to-treat analysis found efficacy in 61% of sacral nerve stimulation patients and 49% in the standard medical therapy group. Adverse events were reported to be 30.5% device-related events in the sacral nerve stimulation group and 27.3% medication-related events in the medical therapy group. In another study, long-term results in 96 patients with refractory overactive bladder were evaluated by voiding diaries.[26] Overall, patients maintained efficacy at mean of 30.8 months (range, 12–60) after implantation in terms of number of incontinence episodes, severity of leakage and number of pads required. Eleven of 96 (11.5%) underwent explant owing to a lack of efficacy, pain, or bowel dysfunction.

Surgery to Treat Stress Urinary Incontinence

Acceptable surgeries to treat stress UI include retropubic urethropexy (modified Burch), pubovesical sling and synthetic midurethral sling. The British guidelines or the National Institute for Health and Care Excellence known as NICE since 2006 have recommended against anterior colporrhaphy, needle suspensions, paravaginal defect repair and the Marshall-Marchetti-Krantz procedure for the treatment of stress UI.[27] The Burch urethropexy or "Burch" involves entering the retropubic space via open incision or laparoscopy and applying sutures to elevate or support the pubovesical tissue to the Cooper's ligament along the inner surface of the pubic bone. A pubovesical sling is performed using a vaginal or combined vaginal/abdominal approach and may implant autologous fascia, harvested from the patient's own rectus (lower abdomen), or fascia lata (outer thigh); allogenic fascia from cadaveric donors; or biologic exogenous implants. A synthetic midurethral sling, or simply a "midurethral sling," involves implantation of a suburethral sling placed at the midurethra, with sling arms placed retropubically in a "U-shape" or through the obturator approach, often referred to as a transobturator sling. Presently, available synthetic slings are composed of type I monofilament polypropylene.

A multicenter randomized, controlled trial that randomized women planning surgery for stress UI to a Burch versus a fascial sling is referred to as the SISTEr trial (Stress Incontinence Surgical Treatment Efficacy Trial).[28] Six hundred sixty-five women were enrolled and 520 completed final assessment at 2 years of follow-up. Success rates for relief in terms of stress UI symptoms was 66% for the fascial sling and 49% for the Burch. However, there were more complications in the sling group with 19 women undergoing 20 procedures to reduce voiding dysfunction or to treat urinary retention. Longer term results have been published on this cohort of patients. Continence rates decreased at 5 years to 30.8% in the sling and 24.1% for the Burch group but satisfaction remained fairly high in both groups.[29] By 7 years, continence rates further declined to 27% in the fascial sling group and 13% for the Burch.[30] Some of the factors associated with lower long-term success were age, menopausal status, prior continence surgery, and recruiting site.

The Ford 2015 Cochrane review of sling surgery of published data on midurethral slings found 81 acceptable trials involving 12,113 women.[31] The conclusions included that midurethral slings are highly effective in the short and medium term and there is increasing evidence of long-term safety. The obturator approach is associated with lower rates of adverse events, except for groin pain. There is not sufficient evidence to find preference for the outside-in or inside-out approach. In terms of the retropubic midurethral sling, there is evidence that the bottom-up approach is superior to top-down. Finally, "mid-urethral sling operations have been the most extensively researched surgical treatment for stress UI in women and have a good safety profile."

The American Urogynecologic Society joint statement with the Society for Female Urology and Urodynamics of January 2014, with reaffirmation in 2015 iterated that:

Polypropylene material is safe and effective as a surgical implant; The monofilament polypropylene mesh midurethral sling is the most extensively studied anti-incontinence procedure in history; Polypropylene mesh midurethral slings are the standard of care for the surgical treatment of SUI & represent a great advance in the treatment of this condition for our patients; The FDA has clearly stated that the polypropylene midurethral sling is safe and effective in the treatment of SUI.[32]

PELVIC ORGAN PROLAPSE

POP refers to the abnormal descent of pelvic organs from their normal attachment sites and into an abnormal position in the pelvis. Prolapse can involve:

- The apical compartment (uterine or vaginal vault prolapse),
- The anterior vaginal wall (cystocele, urethrocele), or
- The posterior compartment (rectocele, enterocele).

Age, vaginal parity higher than 3, and menopause are risk factors associated with symptomatic POP.[33] Other factors such as obesity, chronic heavy lifting, constipation, and genetics are likely contributors. The most common presenting symptom is pressure or bulge.[34] Overwhelmingly, most women with symptoms present with stage II prolapse. Further, most women feel symptoms of POP when the leading edge reaches 0.5 cm distal to the hymenal ring.[35]

Assessment of Pelvic Organ Prolapse

Describing prolapse has been a somewhat controversial issue over the past few decades. Baden-Walker described the half-way system that described the severity of prolapse (anterior, posterior, apical) on a 4-point grading system, with grade 0 indicating perfect support; grade 1 with leading edge "half-way" down the vagina; grade 2 to the introitus; and grade 3 as "half-way" through the hymenal ring and grade 4 as complete prolapse.[36] In an attempt to better quantify location of prolapse and degree for more objective comparison of research outcomes, the International Continence Society in collaboration with American Urogynecologic Society and the Society of Gynecologic Surgeons, created the Pelvic Organ Prolapse Quantification system or the POP-Q. This system used a 9-point measurement system in centimeters including points along the anterior and posterior vaginal walls, the cervix and/or apex, the genital hiatus, and the perineal body.[37] Although more objective than the half-way system, the measurements are cumbersome and largely a research tool. A compromise system that describes the leading edge in centimeters above or below the hymenal ring is more clinically applicable, for example, cervix to +3 cm for a uterine prolapse with the cervix protruding down to 3 cm past the introitus.

Conservative Treatment of Pelvic Organ Prolapse

The general options for treating POP have not changed much over the years. All patients should be offered: observation, vaginal pessary, or surgery. Pelvic floor physical therapy is also a consideration and can help to reduce the degree of prolapse and improve bothersome symptoms. A very recent study compared the cost effectiveness of a vaginal pessary to pelvic floor muscle training in older women with symptomatic prolapse. Both reduced symptoms, yet pessaries did so to a greater degree. Pessaries were found to be more cost effective with the important caveat that many women cannot be successfully fit with a pessary and that pessary use results in more side effects and more office visits.[38]

Younger women who are more active physically and who are sexually active are less likely to find pessaries acceptable, but some definitely will. Thus, pessaries can be offered to all women with symptomatic prolapse. Even if surgery is the ultimate goal, a pessary may provide symptom relief if surgery will not be performed in a timely fashion, or to help a patient decide how reduction of prolapse will change her symptoms.

The most commonly used pessaries in general practice are the Ring pessary, the Gellhorn and the Donut pessary. Choosing the proper pessary size is done manually, similarly to performing a cervical examination on a woman in labor. During digital examination, an estimation of the depth and width with fingers spread without causing patient discomfort. The ring is the easiest to remove and replace and, therefore, preferred first choice if it can be retained. In addition, the ring can remain in place during sexual intercourse. Some women will opt to remove and care for the pessary themselves, whereas others will be unwilling or physically unable to remove a pessary owing to mobility issues. The Gellhorn works through a suction effect and thus may be effective when a ring pessary cannot be retained.[39] The donut pessary provides a space-occupying effect that may provide better relief if incomplete bladder emptying is a main symptom. Rarely will women be able to perform self-care with any pessary other than the ring.

Although the most recent Cochrane review found 1 randomized, controlled trial comparing 2 types of pessaries: the ring and the Gellhorn, they concluded that there is no consensus on best type of pessary or follow-up care.[40] This lack of data extends to use of vaginal estrogen, vaginal antibiotic cream, acidifying ointment, how often to remove and clean a pessary, or when to dispose of a used pessary and replace with a new device. Patients may opt to remove pessaries daily, but vaginal ulcerations, basically caused by pressure, are managed by pessary removal until the ulcer heals. Topical estrogen may hasten ulcer resolution. How long to trial a pessary or how many pessaries to try is a decision made between clinician and the individual patient. When a woman who wears a pessary chronically opts to undergo surgery, assessment of degree of prolapse should be performed when the pessary has been removed and left out for a minimum of 3 days because the full extent of the prolapse may not be readily apparent immediately after pessary removal.

Pelvic Organ Prolapse Surgery

Estimates for the lifetime risk of undergoing prolapse repair surgery range from 11% to 19%.[41,42] Of course, many more women experience symptomatic prolapse than those who opt for surgical solutions, so these numbers underestimate the incidence of POP. There are 4 major decisions to be made when choosing the surgical procedure:

1. Vaginal versus abdominal route (open, laparoscopic, or robotically assisted) or some combination thereof;
2. Hysterectomy versus uterine preservation;
3. Native tissue repair versus mesh augmentation; and
4. Concomitant performance of an incontinence procedure.

As far as route of surgery, a 2010 Cochrane review examining POP surgery concluded that abdominal sacrocolpopexy is associated with lower rate of recurrence than vaginal sacrospinous repair, but in exchange for a longer operative time, recovery time, and cost.[43] An additional conclusion was that continence procedure at time of prolapse surgery in dry women remains controversial.

Traditionally, surgical route and choice of procedure has been based on surgeon experience and comfort. However, data-driven decisions will likely guide decisions in the future. The decision by a gynecologist to perform the prolapse surgery or refer the patient elsewhere should include consideration of his or her ability to assess each compartment (anterior, apical, posterior, and perineum) for defects, and the skill to surgically correct each of these areas, as well as resources available in the community.

No strong data exist to drive decisions regarding hysterectomy versus uterine preservation. Decision making may include surgeon and patient preference, degree of uterine prolapse, plans for future childbearing, and condition of uterus in terms of fibroids, adenomyosis, presence of dysmenorrhea or excessive menstrual bleeding, postmenopausal bleeding, or a markedly elongated cervix.

Vaginally placed mesh remains controversial, especially in the public eye, but increasing scientific data support its safety and efficacy when used in the appropriate patient. The most recent conclusions drawn by the SGS Systematic Review Group were that in the anterior compartment (cystocele repair with mesh augmentation), both anatomic and symptomatic results were better than native tissue repair. There was no benefit to biologic graft in any compartment. Although mesh erosion or exposure occurred in up to 36% of patients, the mesh-related reoperation rates were low and ranged from 3% to 8%.[44] In a recent retrospective review of nearly 5500 surgeries using vaginally placed mesh with a mean follow-up of 5.4 years, overall reoperation for mesh-related complications was 4%. However, in surgeons who performed more than 14 such surgeries per year, the rate was 2% compared with 4.8% for low-volume surgeons. The authors also found that younger age, concomitant hysterectomy, blood transfusion, and medical comorbidities also associated with an increased risk of reoperation.[45] The American College of Obstetricians and Gynecologists Committee Opinion on vaginally placed synthetic mesh stated that mesh should be reserved for high-risk individuals, described as those with recurrent prolapse or medical comorbidities that may add unacceptable risk for open or laparoscopic approaches.[46] This Committee Opinion further recommends that surgeons implanting vaginal mesh ought to have experience with reconstructive surgery and a thorough understanding of the involved pelvic anatomy.

In terms of deciding whether to perform a concomitant incontinence procedure at the time of prolapse surgery, in women who do not experience bothersome preoperative incontinence remains controversial.

The conclusions reached on the management of urethral support at the time of abdominal sacroColpopexy cannot be applied to vaginal repair of prolapse. A Cochrane review concluded that incontinence surgery at time of prolapse repair in dry women remains controversial.[47]

SUMMARY

Many women experience urogynecologic or pelvic floor disorders, especially UI and POP. The OB/GYN is often the first health care professional who will have an opportunity to listen, evaluate, and treat these disorders. A wide variety of treatments are available to treat incontinence, including pelvic floor muscle training, behavioral therapies, oral medications, neuromodulation, intradetrusor medications, and surgery. When approaching the woman with symptomatic prolapse, familiarity with pessaries, and various surgical procedures will aid in counseling the patient appropriately. Referral to a pelvic floor physical therapist or to a female pelvic medicine and reconstructive surgeon should be strongly considered if available and if in the patient's best interests. Increasing attention to data on cost effectiveness is a necessity.

REFERENCES

1. Thom D. Variation in estimates of urinary incontinence prevalence in the community: effects of differences in definition, population characteristics, and study type. J Am Geriatr Soc 1998;46(4):473–80.
2. Nygaard I, Bradley C, Brandt D, Women's Health Initiative. Pelvic organ prolapse in older women: prevalence and risk factors. Obstet Gynecol 2004;104(3):489–97.
3. Haylen BT, De Ridder D, Freeman RM, et al. An International Urogynecological Association (IUGA)/International Continence Society (ICS) joint report on the terminology for female pelvic floor dysfunction. Int Urogynecol J 2010;21(1):5–26.
4. Brink CA, Sampsell CM, Wells TJ, et al. A digital test for pelvic muscle strength in women with urinary incontinence. Nurs Res 1994;43(6):352–6.
5. Laycock J, Jerwood D. Development of the Bradford perineometer. Physiotherapy 1994;80:139–42.
6. Moen MD, Noone MB, Vassallo BJ, et al, Urogynecology Network. Pelvic floor muscle function in women presenting with pelvic floor disorders. Int Urogynecol J Pelvic Floor Dysfunct 2009;20(7):843–6.
7. Lobel RW, Sand PK. The empty supine stress test as a predictor of intrinsic urethral sphincter dysfunction. Obstet Gynecol 1996;88(1):128–32.
8. Haylen BT, Lee J, Logan J, et al. Immediate postvoid residual volumes in women with symptoms of pelvic floor dysfunction. Obstet Gynecol 2008;111(6):1305–12.
9. American Urogynecologic Society (AUGS). AUGS position statement on urodynamics. Available at: http://www.augs.org/index.php?mo=cm&op=ld&fid=218. Accessed August 1, 2016.
10. ACOG Practice Bulletin No. 155 Summary: Urinary Incontinence in Women. Obstetrics & Gynecology 2015;126(5):1120–2.
11. Swithinbank L, Hashim H, Abrams P. The effect of fluid intake on urinary symptoms in women. J Urol 2005;174(1):187–9.
12. Subak LL, Wing R, West DS, et al. Weight loss to treat urinary incontinence in overweight and obese women. PRIDE Investigators. N Engl J Med 2009;360:481–90.
13. Charach G, Greenstein A, Rabinovich P, et al. Alleviating constipation in the elderly improves lower urinary tract symptoms. Gerontology 2001;47:72–6.
14. Coyne KS, Cash B, Kopp C, et al. The prevalence of chronic constipation and faecal incontinence among men and women with symptoms of overactive bladder. BJU Int 2011;107(2):254–61.
15. Phelan L, Kanaya AM, Subak LL, et al. Weight loss prevents urinary incontinence in women with type 2 diabetes: results from the look AHEAD trial. J Urol 2012;187(3):939–44.
16. Danforth KN, Townsend MK, Curhan GC, et al. Type 2 diabetes mellitus and risk of stress, urge and mixed urinary incontinence. J Urol 2009;181(1):193–7.
17. Dumoulin C, Hay-Smith J. Pelvic floor muscle training versus no treatment for urinary incontinence in women. A Cochrane systematic review. Eur J Phys Rehabil Med 2008;44(1):47–63.
18. Richardson ML, Sokol ER. A cost-effectiveness analysis of conservative versus surgical management for the initial treatment of stress urinary incontinence. Am J Obstet Gynecol 2014;211(5):565.e1-6.
19. Staskin D, Kay G, Tannenbaum C, et al. Trospium chloride has no effect on memory testing and is assay undetectable in the central nervous system of older patients with overactive bladder. Int J Clin Pract 2010;64(9):1294–300.

20. Nitti VW, Auerbach S, Martin N, et al. Results of a randomized phase III trial of mirabegron in patients with overactive bladder. J Urol 2013;189(4):138801395.
21. American Urological Association (AUA). Diagnosis and treatment algorithm: AUA/SUFU guideline on non-neurogenic overactive bladder in adults. Available at: http://www.auanet.org/common/pdf/education/clinical-guidance/Overactive-Bladder-Algorithm.pdf. Accessed August 1, 2016.
22. Gaziev G, Topazio L, locovelli V, et al. Percutaneous tibial nerve stimulation (PTNS) efficacy in the treatment of lower urinary tract dysfunctions: a systematic review. BMC Urol 2013;13:61.
23. Peters KM, Carrico DJ, Perez-Marrero RA, et al. Randomized trial of percutaneous tibial nerve stimulation versus sham efficacy in the treatment of overactive bladder syndrome: results from the SUmiT trial. J Urol 2010;183(4):1438–43.
24. Dmochowski R, Chapple C, Nitti VW, et al. Efficacy and safety of onabotulinumtoxinA for idiopathic overactive bladder: a double-blind, placebo controlled, randomized, dose ranging trial. J Urol 2010;184(6):2416–22.
25. Siegel S. Results of a prospective, randomized, multicenter study evaluating sacral neuromodulation with InterStim therapy compared to standard medical therapy at 6-months in subjects with mild symptoms of overactive bladder. Neurourol Urodyn 2015;34:224–40.
26. Janknegt RA, Hassouna MM, Siegel SW, et al. Long-term effectiveness of sacral nerve stimulation for refractory urge incontinence. Eur Urol 2001;39:101–6.
27. National Institute for Health and Care Excellence (NICE). Surgical approaches for SUI. NICE guidance. 2017. Available at: https://www.nice.org.uk/guidance/cg171/chapter/1-recommendations. Accessed August 1, 2016.
28. Albo ME, Richter HE, Brubaker L, et al. Burch colposuspension versus fascial sling to reduce urinary stress incontinence. N Engl J Med 2007;356:2143–55.
29. Brubaker L, Richter HE, Norton PA, et al. 5-year continence rates, satisfaction and adverse events of Burch urethropexy and fascial sling surgery for urinary incontinence. J Urol 2012;187(4):1324–30.
30. Richter HL, Brubaker L, Stoddard AM, et al. Patient related factors associated with long-term urinary continence after Burch colposuspension and pubovaginal fascial sling surgeries. J Urol 2012;188(2):485–9.
31. Ford AA, Rogerson L, Cody JD, et al. Mid-urethral sling operations for stress urinary incontinence in women. Cochrane Database Syst Rev 2015;(7):CD006375.
32. American Urogynecologic Society (AUGS)/Society of Urodynamics and Female Urology (SUFU). AUGS/SUFU position statement on mesh midurethral slings for stress urinary incontinence. Available at: http://www.augs.org/p/bl/et/blogaid=192. Accessed August 1, 2016.
33. Kim CM, Jeon MJ, Chung DJ, et al. Risk factors for pelvic organ prolapse. Int J Gynaecol Obstet 2007;98:248–51.
34. Elkerkman RM, Cundiff GW, Melick CF, et al. Correlation of symptoms with location and severity of prolapse. Am J Obstet Gynecol 2001;185(6):1332–8.
35. Gutman RE, Ford DE, Queroz LH, et al. Is there a pelvic organ prolapse threshold that predicts pelvic floor symptoms? Am J Obstet Gynecol 2008;199(6):683.e1-7.
36. Baden W, Walker T. Surgical repair of vaginal defects. Philadelphia: Lippincott; 1992.
37. Bump RC, Mattiasson A, Bo K, et al. The standardization of terminology of female pelvic organ prolapse and pelvic floor dysfunction. Am J Obstet Gynecol 1996;175(1):10–7.
38. Panman CM, Wiergersma M, Kollen BJ, et al. Effectiveness and cost-effectiveness of pessary treatment compared with pelvic floor muscle training

in older women with pelvic organ prolapse: a 2-year follow-up of a randomized controlled trial in primary care. Menopause 2016;23(12):1307–18.

39. Culligan PJ. Nonsurgical management of pelvic organ prolapse. Obstet Gynecol 2012;119:852–60.
40. Bugge C, Adams EJ, Gopinath D, et al. Pessaries (mechanical devices) for pelvic organ prolapse in women. Cochrane Database Syst Rev 2013;(2):CD004010.
41. Fialkow M, Newton K, Lentz G. Lifetime risk of surgical management for pelvic organ prolapse or urinary incontinence. Int Urogynecol J 2008;19:437–40.
42. Smith FJ, Holman CD, Moorin RE, et al. Lifetime risk of undergoing surgery for pelvic organ prolapse. Obstet Gynecol 2010;116(5):1096–100.
43. Maher CM, Feiner B, Baessler K, et al. Surgical management of pelvic organ prolapse in women: the updated summary version Cochrane review. Int Urogynecol J 2011;22:1445.
44. Schmipf MA, Abed H, Sanses T, et al. Graft and mesh use in transvaginal prolapse repair: a systematic review. Obstet Gynecol 2016;128(1):81–91.
45. Kelly EC, Winick-Ng J, Welk B. Surgeon experience and complications of transvaginal prolapse mesh. Obstet Gynecol 2016;128(1):65–72.
46. Committee Opinion No. 513: Vaginal Placement of Synthetic Mesh for Pelvic Organ Prolapse. Obstetrics & Gynecology 2011;118(6):1459–64.
47. ACOG Committee Opinion No. 444: Choosing the Route of Hysterectomy for Benign Disease. Obstetrics & Gynecology 2009;114(5):1156–8.

The Menopausal Transition

Janice L. Bacon, MD, FACOG

KEYWORDS

- Menopause • Perimenopause • Hormones

KEY POINTS

- Symptoms of menopause often begin 4 to 6 years before the cessation of menses and persist for years.
- Loss of ovarian hormones has widespread and often adverse effects on many organ systems.
- Therapy for menopausal symptoms must be individualized.

Menopause occurs when the ovaries have complete (or near-complete) follicular exhaustion, resulting in very low serum levels of estradiol and markedly increased follicle-stimulating hormone (FSH) levels. Common symptoms of menopause (**Box 1**) often begin during the perimenopausal transition at a median of 47 years or 4 to 6 years before menopause occurs. Because other medical disorders which occur frequently with aging exhibit some of the same symptoms as those of menopause, women may have difficulty distinguishing when they enter the menopausal transition-.This is also true for women who have had irregular menses, an endometrial ablation or a hysterectomy. Symptoms continue for several years after menopause and some women continue to have vasomotor symptoms for even longer periods of time. Almost all women with an intact uterus experience menstrual irregularity in the menopausal transition years resulting from hormonal fluctuations before ovarian follicular depletion.

The largest longitudinal study of women's endocrine and clinical manifestations of menopausal transition comes from the Study of Women's Health Across the Nation (SWAN).[1] This research evaluated and followed more than 3000 women from diverse communities, aged 42 to 52 years, for 15 years. Scientific areas of study for SWAN included bone mineral density and body composition, cardiovascular measures and risk factors, and ovarian markers. Ovarian aging was assessed by serial assessment of FSH, luteinizing hormone, estradiol (E2), inhibin-B, and estrone (E1). Inhibins are peptides of the transforming growth factor family and are produced by granulosa cells of the ovarian follicle. Inhibin levels decline during menopause because of the negative

Disclosure: No disclosure relevant to this topic.
Women's Health and Diagnostic Center, 2728 Sunset Boulevard, Lexington Medical Park 1, Suite 106, West Columbia, SC 29169, USA
E-mail address: jlbacon@lexhealth.org

Obstet Gynecol Clin N Am 44 (2017) 285–296
http://dx.doi.org/10.1016/j.ogc.2017.02.008
0889-8545/17/© 2017 Elsevier Inc. All rights reserved.

obgyn.theclinics.com

Box 1
Frequent symptoms of menopause
Hot flashes (flushes)[a]
Irregular menstrual bleeding
Insomnia
Mood changes (anxiety, depression)
Mastodynia
Headache
Vaginal dryness
[a]Most frequent.

feedback of increasing FSH levels. Other hormonal assays included thyroid-stimulating hormone, dehydroepiandrosterone sulfate (DHEAS), sex hormone–binding globulin, and testosterone.

Results from these cohort studies assisted in defining a staging system now considered the gold standard for characterizing reproductive aging. This staging system, The Stages of Reproductive Aging Workshop (STRAW), in 2001 defined 7 stages of adult women's lives broadly into 3 categories (reproductive, menopausal transition, and postmenopause) with subcategories in each defined by menstrual cycle data and endocrine studies (**Table 1**). In 2011, a review of significant advances in knowledge allowed recommendations for updating criteria and modifying the staging system. Although this system is important for research in maturing women's health, it has applicability also to clinical care in the areas of fertility, contraception, and hormonal therapy.

THE LATE REPRODUCTIVE YEARS

Menstrual cycles are regular, but fertility begins to decline. While cycles are mainly ovulatory, luteal phase progesterone levels decline and the follicular phase becomes

Table 1		
Staging of reproductive aging		
The Late Reproductive Years	**Menopausal Transition (Perimenopause)**	**Menopause**
Regular menses	Varying menstrual intervals	Vasomotor symptoms likely
Declining fertility	Rare fertility	Increased somatic aging
↓ Menstrual intervals	Onset of menopausal symptoms	↓ Estradiol
↓ Luteal phase progesterone	↓ Inhibin-B	↑ FSH
Shortened follicular phase	Variable or ↑ FSH	↓ AMH
Decreasing inhibin-B	↓ AMH	↓↓ Antral follicle count
Normal estradiol	↓ Antral follicle count	
Slightly ↑ FSH		
↓ AMH		
↓ Antral follicle count		

Abbreviation: AMH, antimüllerian hormone.

shorter shorten from 14 to 10 days, resulting in reduced menstrual intervals. This process frequently occurs in the early 40s. Endocrine changes include decreasing inhibin-B and slightly increased FSH levels with preserved levels of estradiol. Antimüllerian hormone (AMH) levels and ovarian antral follicle count decrease.

MENOPAUSAL TRANSITION (PERIMENOPAUSE)

In the early phase of perimenopause, menstrual intervals begin to vary by 7 days or more in consecutive cycles. In addition, there accompanying change in FSH levels, which are variable to increased. AMH and inhibin-B levels remain low.

The late phase of menopausal transition occurs 1 to 3 years before cessation of menses and is characterized by increased menstrual intervals of more than 60 days. FSH levels are increased ($\geq$25 IU/L) with low AMH level, antral follicle count (AFC), and inhibin-B level. Vasomotor symptoms are regularly reported.

MENOPAUSE

For about 2 years after the final menstrual period, vasomotor symptoms are the most likely. These symptoms correspond with persistent increased FSH levels, low AMH and inhibin-B levels, and very low antral follicle count. Estradiol levels continue to decrease and FSH levels to increase for about 2 years after the final menses. Then for the next 3 to 6 years FSH stabilizes and FSH, AMH, and inhibin-B levels are all very low.

These first 1 to 6 years after the final menses are now termed early menopause. Following these years, vasomotor symptoms persist in some women but are less likely and symptoms of urogenital atrophy are more notable. Somatic aging processes are more marked.

The demographic factors of body mass index (BMI), chronologic age, demographic factors, and lifestyle may influence reproductive aging; however, research using epidemiologic and clinical information shows a predictable pattern for most women. Factors of BMI and smoking may influence the timing of changes but not the "trajectory of change in bleeding patterns or hormonal levels with reproductive aging."[2] This process does not apply to women undergoing premature ovarian failure, likely because of the varied causes and possible resumption of menses and ability to conceive.

Some other medical conditions or a history of endometrial ablation or hysterectomy affect the prediction of transition. Women with amenorrhea from endometrial ablation, or who have had a hysterectomy, can only be assessed by endocrine markers of ovarian aging. Because surgery may result in a transient increase of FSH level, accurate endocrine levels may not be achieved for at least 3 months postoperativley. For a firm diagnosis, a single serum estradiol or FSH result may need to be repeated.[3,4]

Polycystic ovary syndrome is commonly associated with oligomenorrhea and therefore use of bleeding patterns is less reliable when assessing reproductive aging. Menstrual criteria are also not useful in endocrine disorders with an increased incidence of amenorrhea, such as hypothalamic amenorrhea. Information about the transition to menopause is needed for women with these disorders. Medications, chronic illness, or loss of significant amounts of body fat may also affect menstrual patterns and eliminate the use of bleeding patterns to assist in determining menopause.

Women undergoing treatment of malignancy may experience months of amenorrhea and symptoms of menopause. Age at treatment and use of chemotherapeutic agents may also influence menopausal timing. Alkylating agents especially may lead to transient increases of FSH levels and decreased AMH and AFC but with time

(12 months or more) menses may resume.[5-7] Resumption of menstrual bleeding may not indicate normal menstrual function. In women being treated with tamoxifen, assessment of menopause may also be difficult, because this medication may alter FSH and estradiol levels and, because of its effects on the endometrium, may cause abnormal bleeding.[8]

Predicting the final menstrual period (FMP) is important for considering bone density loss and cardiovascular risks, because these risks begin to increase in the year before the FMP. Use of FSH and AMH levels as well as AFC combined with age and other factors such as BMI are under study to develop a method to more accurately anticipate this event. Because ovulatory cycles can occur until 12 months of amenorrhea have occurred, contraception should be a part of any discussion during the menopausal transition.

In addition to the hormonal changes described in the hypothalamic-pituitary-ovarian axis, adrenal changes during the menopausal transition are associated with increases in serum cortisol levels accompanied by transient increases in levels of adrenal androgens (androstenediol, dehydroepiandrosterone sulfate, and others). No specific changes in thyroid function related to menopause have been identified.

After menopause, the greatest estrogen production is from aromatization of androgens in the ovarian stroma and, to a lesser extent, from production in extragonadal sites, including adipose tissue, muscle, bone, bone marrow, fibroblasts, and hair roots.[9] Most of the aromatization of androgens to estrogen takes place in adipose tissue.

SYMPTOMS AND PHYSICAL CHANGES OF MENOPAUSE
Vasomotor Symptoms

The most well-described symptom of menopause is the hot flash, or hot flush, a vasomotor symptom that occurs in up to 80% of women. These flashes may begin during the late reproductive years but are generally mild and may be associated with menses, but after the FMP their frequency and intensity increase greatly. Nocturnal events are often described as night sweats. The most common description of the event is a sudden onset of a feeling of heat in the face or upper chest, which may continue there or become more generally perceived throughout the body. The duration is often 2 to 4 minutes and the feeling is accompanied by varying amounts of perspiration. Additional symptoms include flushing of the face, neck, and upper chest; palpitations; and anxiety. It may be followed at times by chills and shivering. They may be particularly disturbing at night, disrupting sleep and requiring changes of clothing or bedclothes. The frequency ranges from 1 to 2 per day up to 1 or more per hour.[10,11] These continue for more than a year in 80% of women but commonly abate in 4 to 5 years without treatment. However, up to 9% of women continue to experience them for many years.

Obese women often report more significant or frequent vasomotor symptoms. Although a popular belief is that menopause is associated with weight gain, in reality weight gain is more associated with aging and lifestyle changes.

Recently new research has begun to link a history of experiencing large numbers of hot flashes to markers of cardiovascular risk, noting that some frequent hot flashes may identify a vulnerable vascular phenotype.[12]

Some specific triggers for hot flashes include drinking hot liquids, moving quickly into an environment with a different temperature, and spicy foods. Symptoms that significantly disrupt daily life warrant a discussion of therapeutic options. Many therapies, medical and nonmedical, have been tried with varying results to assist symptom management (**Boxes 2** and **3**).

Box 2
Therapeutic options for vasomotor symptoms

Menopausal hormone therapy

Selective estrogen receptor modulator (SERM; bazedoxifene and conjugated estrogens)

Lifestyle changes
    Weight Loss
    Environmental temperature
    Smoking cessation
    Exercise
    Relaxation techniques

Dietary supplements
    Soy products
    Isoflavone supplements
    Black cohosh
    Vitamin E
    Omega-3
    Fatty acids

Selective serotonin reuptake inhibitors

Serotonin/norepinephrine reuptake inhibitors

Gabapentin

Clonidine

Compounded hormone therapy

Alternative therapies
  Acupuncture, hypnosis

Sleep Disturbance

Women undergoing the menopause transition are at increased risk for loss of quality sleep, and vasomotor symptoms may additionally disrupt sleep. These symptoms may produce chronic insomnia, which, with time, has effects on overall well-being, health, and productivity.[13]

In addition, common sleep disorders, such as sleep apnea, restless legs, and other forms of insomnia, increase in incidence in women of menopausal age. Depression also increases in midlife women and disordered sleep is a common symptom of depression and anxiety.[14]

Treatment of vasomotor symptoms by lifestyle changes, supplements, or prescription therapies, as well as therapy for other sleep disorders, relieves these symptoms and improves quality of life. Failure to relieve insomnia should lead to formal sleep studies, because pharmacologic sleep medications are for short-term use only.

Headache

Although the causes of headache are many and tension headaches are the most common headache, hormonally related migraine headaches may increase in the menopausal transition because of hormonal fluctuations. After menopause, symptoms often decrease again, but migraine headaches with aura convey a significant increased risk for stroke, particularly for women who smoke. Migraine headache with aura may show less improvement after menopause than migraine headache without aura. New onset of headaches in women more than 50 years

---

Box 3
Menopausal hormone therapy

Systemic therapy

Estrogen alone
  Conjugated estrogens (equine or synthetic)
  Esterified estrogens, estropipate
  Micronized 17B estradiol
  Ethinyl estradiol, estradiol acetate

Delivery routes: oral, transdermal (vaginal ring, spray or gel or cream, patch), implants

Progestogen therapy[a]

Micronized progesterone: oral, injectable; Medroxyprogesterone acetate: oral or depomedroxyprogesterone; Norethindrone, norethindrone acetate: oral; Progesterone gel: transdermal; Levonorgestrel intrauterine system; Norgestrel: oral; Megestrol acetate: oral

Combined estrogen and progestogen: oral transdermal patch

Combined estrogen/methyltestosterone: oral

Selective estrogen receptor modulator (SERM)

Ospemifene; Bazedoxifene (formulated with conjugated estrogens); Raloxifene

Local estrogen therapy

Estrogen (vaginal)
  17B estradiol: cream
  Estradiol: tablet
  Estradiol acetate: ring
  Conjugated estrogens: cream

DHEA vaginal ovules

[a]Combined with an estrogen in patients with an intact uterus.

---

old, worst-ever headache, sudden-onset headaches with activity or nocturnal awakening, or those with neurologic manifestations should prompt thorough investigation.

Tension headaches often respond well to use of nonsteroidal therapies or to prevention with tricyclic antidepressants rather than hormone therapy alone. Hormone therapy for vasomotor symptoms is satisfactory for women with tension or migraine headaches. Noncyclic therapies are recommended to minimize hormonally triggered headache. Women with migraine headache without aura and who have not yet reached menopause may benefit from monophasic oral contraceptives (if no other contraindications exist). Those women with migraine headache with aura or other risk factors for stroke may benefit from progestin-only therapies such as a levonorgestrel-containing intrauterine device, etonogestrel contraceptive implant, depomedroxyprogesterone acetate, or progesterone-only oral contraceptives.

Cognition and Mood

Patient complaints of poor memory are common during the menopausal transition and early menopause, but commonly improve after early menopause and return to normal unless other medical disorders arise. Symptoms include reduced concentration and slower mental performance. Expression of symptoms may be affected by sleep, mental health disorders, medications, or life stressors.

Estrogen may slow the rate of decline of memory function.[15,16] The Women's Health Initiative (WHI) did not show a positive effect of estrogen on cognitive function, but women with surgical menopause before age 50 years may be prescribed estrogen to decrease the risk of dementia later in life. Estrogen may reduce the risk or delay the onset of Alzheimer disease, although no role for estrogen in the treatment of Alzheimer has been shown.[17,18] In contrast, estrogen therapy initiation after age 65 years could increase the risk of dementia. Because dementia and cognitive decline may be related to cardiovascular disease, women with these concerns should be referred for evaluation of systemic disease.

Women may complain of low mood or mood swings during menopausal transition. New-onset depression may occur during the menopausal transition and the diagnosis occurs less often after menopause.[19,20] Because of the ages of women commonly going through menopause transition, these chronologic years are associated with increasing incidence of other medical disorders as well as family and social events, such as becoming so-called empty nesters and caring for aging parents, which contribute potential stressors associated with depressive symptoms. Although hormone therapy may assist in modification of some of these effects, antidepressants or antianxiety medications along with cognitive behavior measures and lifestyle modification (sleep, diet, exercise) may provide the best benefit.

Urogenital Atrophy

Estrogen deficiency early in the menopausal transition may be first recognized by decreased lubrication with arousal and sexual activity. As estrogen levels continue to decrease and as time passes, this effect becomes more marked, sometimes resulting not only in dyspareunia but in dryness with normal activities, resulting in itching and discomfort. Blood flow to the vagina and vulva is reduced, contributing to skin changes. The appearance of the external genitalia reveals less pubic hair and less elasticity of the vulvar skin with introital narrowing and possible changes in architecture, such as loss of the labia minora. Vulvar dystrophies, vulvar lesions or dysplasia, or other dermatologic disorders should be excluded.

Chronic hypoestrogenemia produces visual changes, including thinner more glossy tissue appearance, pale pink coloration, and loss of rugae in the vagina. The elasticity of the vagina lessens and the vagina may become shorter or narrower. Continued sexual function may decrease these changes, even without hormonal therapy. These changes commonly develop around 3 years after menopause, although about 20% of women report some symptoms in the early or late menopause transition.[17] The uterus and any fibroids become smaller and the cervix appears atrophied and may become flush with the vaginal vault. Symptoms of endometriosis and adenomyosis abate. Ovarian size decreases and palpation on examination may be limited.

Urinary tract and vaginal pH changes with resulting alterations in bacterial flora may lead to some itching and malodorous discharge and may contribute to dyspareunia. The possibility of sexually transmitted diseases must not be overlooked in sexually active women with these symptoms. Vaginal atrophy and associated microabrasions occurring with sexual activity may increase the risks of infection if exposed. Women born between 1945 and 1965 are at the highest risks of hepatitis C. Evidence-based guidelines from the Centers for Disease Control and Prevention provide current recommendations for treatment.

Although many women try vaginal lubricants and moisturizers initially, topical estrogen is the best treatment for relief of vulvovaginal symptoms and current therapeutic options for topical administration include vaginal cream or tablet preparations or a vaginal ring.[21] Systemic estrogen preparations with or without progesterone provide excellent vaginal therapy, but may be contraindicated or less desirable to some women. Also available is a daily oral medication, ospemifene, an estrogen receptor antagonist with a side chain that is proestrogen in the vulvar and vaginal tissues. It produces mucosal changes similar to estrogen preparations which increase tissue thickness and lubrication.

Vaginal estrogen may be used in women undergoing therapy for cancer of the breast, those using tamoxifen, or those who have completed therapy and are experiencing genitourinary symptoms on nonhormonal therapies. Less information regarding women using aromatase inhibitors is available because initiation of vaginal estrogen initially increases serum estrogen levels, but the increase is not maintained and overall levels remain low. Although the vaginal ring or tablet may produce the most consistent dosing, creams also provide a very low dose of estrogen to the vaginal tissues when dosed appropriately. Fewer data are available on creams containing conjugated estrogens than on those containing 17B-estradiol.[22]

The newest development in topical therapy for vaginal atrophy is an intravaginal preparation of 0.5% dehydroepiandrosterone (DHEA), a nonestrogen hormone produced by the ovary and adrenal glands that can relieve vaginal dryness and painful intercourse.[23] Both ospemifene and DHEA not only provide symptom relief but, like estrogen preparations, produce clinically visible improvement in vaginal appearance, secretions, and thickness. In addition to medical therapies, laser therapy for vaginal tissue has been available, but results are mixed, and this alternative to medical treatment may result in adhesions and vaginal scarring.

Joint and Bone Changes

Joint discomfort increases with increasing age, as does the incidence of rheumatologic disorders. Women who are obese or have depression may have accentuated symptoms. However, there seems to be an association with joint pain and the menopausal transition. These symptoms may be relieved by estrogen therapy alone or combination estrogen/progestin therapy, as noted in the WHI.[24]

Osteopenia and osteoporosis are accelerated in development after menopause, mainly because of accelerated bone resorption, whereas bone formation continues at premenopausal rates. Cortical bone is less affected than trabecular bone, thus this loss of bone is most pronounced in vertebral, coaxial, and radial sites. This rapid rate of loss in late menopause, and for a few years after, exceeds the rate of loss associated with aging and may achieve 20% of lifetime loss.[25] Lifetime risks of fracture after menopause are also affected by the individual's earlier bone density, age at menopause, and other risk factors or medications associated with low bone density. Additional factors include race, smoking status, body habitus, physical activity, serum androgens, and sun exposure. Bone densitometry is the most accurate predictor of bone density, although the age of initiation, frequency of testing and impact of multiple risk factors has not been determined. Fracture risk may also be estimate by FRAX (Fracture Risk Assessment Tool) determination or more elaborate testing, such as dual energy x-ray absorptiometry.

Many treatments are available for use in preventing fractures in menopausal women and both oral and transdermal estrogen therapies are approved for prevention of osteoporosis in at-risk women. A list of therapies for preventing osteoporosis-related fractures is shown in **Box 4**. Estrogens are considered second-line therapies at this time and assist with maintenance of bone density. Androgens have not been studied in women for prevention of bone loss.

Box 4
Treatment options for preventing fractures in women with osteoporosis

Bisphosphonates: prevent loss of bone mass

SERMs: decrease bone resorption

Calcium/vitamin D: increase serum 25-hydroxyvitamin D_3

Calcitonin: inhibits osteoclasts

Estrogen therapy: decreases bone resorption

Systemic hormone preparations: decreases bone resorption

Bazedoxifene (SERM and congugated estrogens): decreases bone resorption

---

CARDIOVASCULAR CHANGES IN MENOPAUSE

Cardiovascular disease (CVD) is the leading cause of death in postmenopausal women. Menopause increases risk for CVD independent of age. Results of the WHI showed that hormone therapy does not prevent CVD. Analysis from the Estrogen-Alone Trial suggested that hormone treatment effects differed by age and that younger women versus their older counterparts had a lower risk of CVD, likely associated with less atherosclerotic development. These effects of greater safety and decreased incidence of disease also applied to overall mortality, colorectal cancer, and global index of disease.[26] The benefit of estrogen on cardiovascular mortality is likely multifactorial: estrogen-related reduction of low-density lipoprotein levels and increase of high-density lipoprotein levels, and improved endothelial function in coronary vasculature.[27]

BREAST CANCER AND MENOPAUSE

The relationship of estrogen to postmenopausal development of breast cancer is controversial and study results regarding causation are mixed. In the WHI study, the incidence of breast cancer increased in the estrogen-progestin arm of the study and decreased in the estrogen-only and placebo arms. These findings continued in the follow-up studies of this population. The slightly increased relative risk of breast cancer could have been related to the length of hormone use or the sequential administration of the progestin therapy or even the progestin formulation itself. In contrast, hormone therapy users had more localized tumors and improved survival rates. Individual risks are very small.

Breast cancer survivors with menopausal symptoms and vulvovaginal atrophy have fewer choices of therapy because systemic therapy is not advised for hormone-dependent tumors. Options for symptom management include nonhormonal moisturizers, vaginal estrogens, androgens, selective estrogen receptor modulators (SERMs), laser therapy, or nonprescription interventions such as acupuncture, dietary supplements, and lifestyle changes. Women using tamoxifen should not use paroxetine for vasomotor symptoms. SERMs may also increase the risk of thrombosis and should be avoided in women with a high risk of thrombosis.

VENOUS THROMBOEMBOLISM

The risks of thromboembolism increase with increased age combined with medical comorbidities. Venous thromboembolism (VTE) is a multifactorial disease with risks increased by decreased mobilization, surgery, malignancy, and medications.

Although the risks of VTE associated with hormonal combined contraceptive use have been widely discussed, the use of menopausal hormonal therapies also increases the risks for VTE. Current use of estrogen preparations alone and estrogen/progestin combination medical regimens increase the risks of VTE 2-fold or 3-fold, with oral combined estrogen/progestin regimens conferring a higher risk than estrogen alone. Transdermal preparations of estrogen or estrogen and progestin combined medication and vaginal estrogen preparations seemed not to increase the VTE risks.[28]

NORTH AMERICAN MENOPAUSE SOCIETY RECOMMENDATIONS

In 2014, the North American Menopause Society (NAMS) released recommendations concerning the clinical care of midlife women. This publication provides an overview of menopause and the physiologic changes followed by a succinct discussion of symptoms of menopausal transition and clinical recommendations for care. Many of the recommendations were discussed earlier in this article.[29] Additional areas discussed in the NAMS publication include:

Skin and Hair

Decreased skin thickness and collagen result in more skin laxity and wrinkling, with symptoms exacerbated by sun and environmental factors and smoking. Many women experience hair loss after completing the menopause transition, whereas others note hirsutism. Testing for women with hair loss includes thyroid function, serum iron, and excluding androgen excess. Loss of ovarian estrogen production results in a relative androgen-excess environment, which may also be influenced by genetic factors and a history of androgen excess. Therapeutic approaches that block peripheral androgens combined with pharmacologic medications or aesthetic procedures for removal of unwanted hair provide the best approach. More study is needed to strengthen the level of recommendations for managing these problems.

Eyes

Menopause is associated with increasing symptoms of dry eyes and cataract development. The initial therapy for dry eyes is topical lubricants and antiinflammatory agents.

Ears

The incidence of hearing loss increases beyond age 50 years. The cause of hearing loss is multifactorial but it may increase social withdrawal and depression. Physiologic levels of estrogen may assist with hearing preservation but estrogen/progestin combination therapy may have a small negative effect.

Teeth and Oral Cavity

Loss of estrogen is associated with thinning and recession of gingival tissue. In addition, low bone mineral density may lead to an increased risk of tooth loss and periodontal disease.

Gallbladder Disease

An increased risk of gallbladder disease has been shown with both estrogen therapy alone and estrogen/progestin combination therapy. The risk of disease seems greater with oral versus transdermal hormone therapy and all systemic hormone therapy should be prescribed with caution to women with known gallbladder disease.

Epilepsy

Menopause may occur earlier in women with epilepsy. The cause could be associated with the number of lifetime seizures or with seizure medications, particularly those metabolized by the hepatic cytochrome P 450 enzyme, which also affects estrogen metabolism and levels. Many women have hormonally sensitive seizures and, during the hormonal fluctuations of the menopause transition, may have an increased number of seizures. Pharmacologic approaches suggested for management include natural progestin supplementation or menstrual suppression with depomedroxyprogesterone acetate or gonadotropin-releasing hormone agonists. In addition, the antiepileptic medication gabapentin may assist with vasomotor symptoms, whereas other seizure medications may accelerate vitamin D metabolism, possibly increasing risks for osteopenia.

The NAMS document also provides recommendations for clinical history, screening for malignancies, as well as clinical evaluation and counseling patients. Both summaries of prescription and nonprescription therapies in menopause and for menopausal symptoms are reviewed.[29]

Perhaps the most important concept in the care of women in the menopausal transition is individual assessment of risks, clinical needs, and symptom relief for the present and for future health and well-being.

REFERENCES

1. Sowers MF, Crawford S, Sternfeld B, et al. SWAN: a multi-center, multi-ethnic, community based cohort study of women and the menopause. In: Lobo R, Marcus R, editors. Menopause: Biology and Pathobiology. San Diego (CA): Academic Press; 2000. p. 175–688.
2. Harlow SD, Gass M, Hall JE, et al. Executive Summary of the States of Reproductive Aging Workshop +10: addressing the unfinished agenda of staging reproductive aging. Menopause 2012;19(4):387–95.
3. Hehenkamp WJ, Volkers NA, Broekmans FJ, et al. Loss of ovarian reserve after uterine artery embolization: a randomized comparison with hysterectomy. Hum Reprod 2007;22:1996–2005.
4. Qu X, Cheng Z, Yang W, et al. Controlled clinical trial assessing the effect of laparoscopic uterine arterial occlusion on ovarian reserve. J Minim Invasive Gynecol 2010;17:47–52.
5. Broekmans FJ, Soules MR, Fauser BC. Ovarian aging: mechanisms and clinical consequences. Endocr Rev 2009;30:465–93.
6. Su HI, Sammel MD, Green J, et al. Antimullerian hormone and inhibin B are hormone measures of ovarian function in late reproductive-aged breast cancer survivors. Cancer 2010;116:592–9.
7. Sukumvanich P, Case LD, Van Zee K, et al. Incidence and time course of bleeding after long-term amenorrhea after breast cancer treatment: a prospective study. Cancer 2010;116:3102–11.
8. Welt CK, Pagan YL, Smith PC, et al. Control of follicle-stimulating hormone by estradiol and the inhibins: critical role of estradiol at the hypothalamus during the luteal-follicular transition. J Clin Endocrinol Metab 2003;88:1766–71.
9. Smith KE, Judd HL. Menopause and postmenopause. In: De Cherney AH, Pernoll ML, editors. Current obstetric and gynecologic diagnosis and treatment. 8th edition. New York: Lange Medical Books; 1994. p. 1030–50.
10. Randolph JF, Sowers M, Bondarenko I, et al. The relationship of longitudinal change in reproductive hormones and vasomotor symptoms during the menopausal transition. J Clin Endocrinol Metab 2005;90:6106.

11. Thurston RC, Joffe H. Vasomotor symptoms and menopause: findings from the Study of Women's Health Across the Nation. Obstet Gynecol Clin North Am 2011;38:489.

12. Thurston RC, Chang Y, Barinas-Mitchell E, et al. Menopausal hot flashes and carotid intima media thickness among midlife women. Stroke 2016;47(12):2910–5.

13. Dennerstein L, Dudley EC, Hopper JL, et al. A prospective population-based study of menopausal symptoms. Obstet Gynecol 2000;96:351.

14. Freedman RR, Roehrs TA. Sleep disturbance in menopause. Menopause 2007; 14:826.

15. Sherwin BB. Estrogen effects on cognition in menopausal women. Neurology 1997;48:S21–6.

16. Resnick SM, Metter EJ, Zonderman AB. Estrogen replacement therapy and longitudinal decline in visual memory. A possible protective effect? Neurology 1997; 49(6):1491–7.

17. Tang MX, Jacobs D, Stern Y, et al. Effect of estrogen during menopause on risk and age at onset of Alzheimer's disease. Lancet 1996;9025:429–32.

18. Kawas C, Resnick S, Morrison A, et al. A prospective study of estrogen replacement therapy and the risk of developing Alzheimer's disease: the Baltimore Longitudinal Study of Aging. Neurology 1997;6:1517–21.

19. Avis NE, Brambilla D, McKinlay SM, et al. A longitudinal analysis of the association between menopause and depression. Results from the Massachusetts Women's Health Study. Ann Epidemiol 1994;4:214.

20. Freeman EW, Sammel MD, Lin H, et al. Associations of hormones and menopausal status with depressed mood in women with no history of depression. Arch Gen Psychiatry 2006;63:375.

21. Suckling JA, Kennedy R, Lethaby A, et al. Local oestrogen for vaginal atrophy in postmenopausal women. Cochrane Database Syst Rev 2006;(4):CD001500.

22. The Use of Vaginal Estrogen in Women With a History of Estrogen-Dependent Breast Cancer. Committee Opinion No. 659, American College of Obstetricians and Gynecologists. March 2016.

23. Labrie F, Archer DF, Koltun W, et al. Efficacy of intravaginal dehydroepiandrosterone (DHEA) on moderate to severe dyspareunia and vaginal dryness, symptoms of vulvovaginal atrophy, and of the genitourinary syndrome of menopause. Menopause 2016;23(3):243–56.

24. Barnabei VM, Cochrane BB, Aragaki AK, et al. Menopausal symptoms and treatment-related effects of estrogen and progestin in the Women's Health Initiative. Obstet Gynecol 2005;105:1063.

25. Grady D, Cummings SR. Postmenopausal hormone therapy for prevention of fractures: how good is the evidence? JAMA 2001;285(22):2909–10.

26. LaCroix AZ, Chlebowski RT, Manson JE, et al. Health outcomes after stopping conjugated equine estrogens among postmenopausal women with prior hysterectomy: a randomized controlled trial. JAMA 2011;305(13):1305–14.

27. Williams JK, Hall J, Anthony MS, et al. A comparison of tibolone and hormone replacement therapy on coronary artery and myocardial function in ovariectomized atherosclerotic monkeys. Menopause 2002;9(1):41–51.

28. Bergendal A, Kieler H, Sundström A, et al. Risk of venous thromboembolism associated with local and systemic use of hormone therapy in peri- and postmenopausal women and in relation to type and route of administration. Menopause 2016;23(6):593–9.

29. Shifren JL, Gass ML. The North American Menopause Society recommendations for clinical care of midlife women. Menopause 2014;21(10):1–25.

Special Article

Burnout in Obstetricians and Gynecologists

Roger P. Smith, MD

KEYWORDS

• Burnout • Depression • Exhaustion • Prevention • Stress

KEY POINTS

- The risk of burnout is ubiquitous, placing all professionals at risk.
- It is estimated that 40% to 75% of obstetricians and gynecologists currently suffer from professional burnout, making the lifetime risk a virtually certainty.
- The spectrum of professional burnout varies from emotional fatigue to complete collapse, substance addiction, and suicidal ideation.
- Several simple strategies can blunt, if not eliminate, the risk of professional burnout.

INTRODUCTION

There just never seems to be enough time to deal with all the directions in which one is pulled; the pace of life, its stresses, the impact of multitasking, and the unending bombardment of information have spiraled out of control. This can easily result in the exhaustion of physical or emotional strength or motivation, otherwise known as *burnout*. Burnout is physical or mental collapse caused by overwork or stress, and all professionals are at risk—loss of control (real or imagined), conflicting demands on time from every direction, and a diminishing sense of worth erodes physician's lives.

It is estimated that 40% to 75% of obstetricians and gynecologists currently suffer from professional burnout, making the lifetime risk a virtually certainty.[1,2] In an online study of more than 15,800 physicians who responded to a survey that included the prevalence of burnout, defined as loss of enthusiasm for work, feelings of cynicism, and a low sense of personal accomplishment, more than one-half of obstetricians and gynecologists demonstrated burnout (**Fig. 1**).[3] Although these statistics make for a dismal view of the profession, if the causes and symptoms can be identified simple steps can be implemented to reverse the threat. With a little care, the enjoyment of practice can be restored and the sense of reward and the value of service can be returned.

Disclosure Statement: The author has nothing to disclose.
Charles E. Schmidt College of Medicine, Florida Atlantic University, 777 Glades Road, BC-71, Room 337, Boca Raton, FL 33431, USA
E-mail address: rogersmith@health.fau.edu

Obstet Gynecol Clin N Am 44 (2017) 297–310
http://dx.doi.org/10.1016/j.ogc.2017.02.006
0889-8545/17/© 2017 Elsevier Inc. All rights reserved.

obgyn.theclinics.com

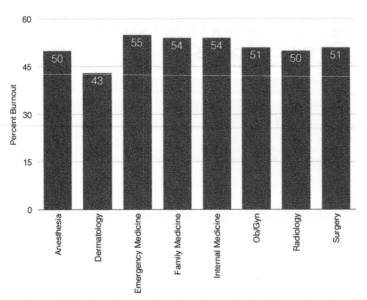

Fig. 1. Prevalence of physician burnout in selected specialties. Selected results of an online survey of more than 15,800 physicians that included the prevalence of burnout (defined as loss of enthusiasm for work, feelings of cynicism, and a low sense of personal accomplishment). (*Adapted from* Medscape Lifestyle Report 2016: bias and burnout. Available at: http://www.medscape.com/features/slideshow/lifestyle/2016/public/overview#page52. Accessed September 16, 2016.)

THE PROBLEM IS PERVASIVE
All Physicians are at Risk

Professional burnout is not new—what is new is the wider recognition of the alarming rates of burnout.[4,5] Physicians, in general, have burnout rates that are twice the rate of working adults, and no area of practice within medicine is immune to the impact of professional burnout (see **Fig. 1**).[1,6] A 2015 survey of plastic surgeons[7] found that nearly one-third (29%) of those surveyed scored high in subscale categories predictive of professional burnout, consistent with other national surveys.[8] In a sample of 127 headache medicine specialists, 66 (57.4%) physicians reported symptoms of professional burnout reflected by high emotional exhaustion or high depersonalization.[9]

A 2015, meta-analysis of burnout in emergency physicians found moderate to high levels of burnout with difficult work conditions including significant psychological demands, lack of resources, and poor support,[10] consistent with older studies that found rates of burnout in excess of 60%.[11] Nonetheless, these physicians reported high job satisfaction. Many pediatric emergency physicians report feeling burned out at work (88.5%) or more callous toward people as a result of work (67.5%) at least monthly, with 1 in 5 reporting such feelings at least weekly.[12] Pediatric intensivists have burnout rates of almost 80%, and a reference group of general pediatricians had an almost 30% rate of emotional exhaustion and depersonalization; this rate was lower for professional accomplishment.[13]

In a study of US surgeons, 40% of those responding were burned out, 30% screened positive for symptoms of depression, and 28% had a mental quality of life score greater than 1/2 standard deviation below the population norm.[14] Almost 50% of anesthesiologists scored positive for burnout domains in different surveys, with one-third reporting high levels.[15] In a 2015 study of US neurosurgeons, the overall burnout rate was 56.7%, and 30% of those surveyed would not choose a career in neurosurgery again.[16]

Physician burnout is not restricted to the United States. In a 2016 study to determine the incidence of burnout among UK and Irish urologic consultants and nonconsultant hospital doctors, high levels of burnout were found, characterized by emotional exhaustion and depersonalization.[17] These were associated with significant levels of self-medication, and 60% reported that they would take advantage of counseling if offered. In a cross-sectional study of Austrian physicians, 10.3% were affected by major depression, and more than 50% of the participants were affected by symptoms of burnout.[18] Among Australian and New Zealand radiation oncologists, nearly half of the respondents scored highly in at least 1 burnout subscale.[19]

The Prevalence in Obstetricians and Gynecologists

A recent survey of gynecologic oncologists[20] found that 30% of study subjects scored high for emotional exhaustion, 10% high for depersonalization, and 11% low for personal accomplishment—all markers for burnout. Overall, almost one-third (32%) of the physicians studied had scores indicating burnout. More concerning was that 33% screened positive for depression, 13% had a history of suicidal ideation, 15% screened positive for alcohol abuse, and 34% reported impaired quality of life. Almost 40% would not encourage their children to enter medicine, and more than 10% said that they would not choose medicine as a career again if they had to do it over.

Although burnout in subspecialists in obstetrics and gynecology has been well documented,[20,21] less well understood is the difference, if any, between those who practice the full scope of obstetrics and gynecology and those who subspecialize. Weinstein,[22] writing in this journal, speculated that practice patterns such as "laborist" may result in fewer stresses of a private practice, with a more predictable and controllable schedule, although a reduction in burnout rates is unreported.

Residents and Young Physicians are at Increased Risk

Although professional burnout can occur at any point in a physician's career, young clinicians are at particular risk, with residents and those at midcareer particularly vulnerable.[23] Resident burnout rates are reported as high as 75%.[3,24] In a 2012 study, of the surveyed residents, 13% satisfied all 3 subscale scores for high burnout and greater than 50% had high levels of depersonalization and emotional exhaustion.[25] Those with high levels of emotional exhaustion were less satisfied with their careers, regretted choosing obstetrics and gynecology, and had higher rates of depression—all consistent with older studies.[26,27]

A study of Australian trainees found a total incidence of burnout of 55.9%, with the highest rates in the first year of training,[28] and among orthopedic trainees, 53% were considered burned out.[29] In another study of 204 doctors undergoing residency training in multiple specialties in a tertiary hospital, 45.6% of respondents reported burnout in the dimension of emotional exhaustion, 57.8% in the dimension of depersonalization, and 61.8% in the dimension of reduced personal accomplishment.[30] The impact of burnout for early to midcareer practitioners is less well studied, but based on the small differences found in studies across students, residents, and early career physicians by Dyrbye and colleagues,[31] it is reasonable to assume that burnout continues to be at least as prevalent in these years.

IDENTIFYING THE CAUSE

In medicine and other professions, the likelihood of burnout happening depends on personal, developmental-psychodynamic, professional, and environmental factors, but the exact role of each in the development of burnout is incompletely understood.[32] The very same attributes that make successful physicians (eg, type-A behavior, obsessive-compulsive commitment to the profession) increase the risk for professional burnout. In general, autonomy, the power to make decisions, the workload, and working hours seem to be the greatest drivers of emotional exhaustion, the strongest predictor of burnout.[33]

Positive depression screening, pathologic sleepiness, and sleeping less than 7 hours a night were independent predictors of burnout in a study of medical students published in 2016.[34] In other studies, a high level of depersonalization has been inversely correlated to job satisfaction and personal accomplishment and strongly correlated to depression—both risk factors for burnout.[25] A high level of personal accomplishment has been strongly correlated with job satisfaction and satisfaction with obstetrics and gynecology as a specialty but was inversely correlated with a sense of depersonalization. No correlation between burnout and self-care activities was found. Similarly, younger age and greater job dissatisfaction have been found to predict higher depersonalization; lower coworker support and greater job dissatisfaction predict lower personal accomplishment.[35]

Unlike earlier studies, a 2016 study found that women were at greater risk of professional burnout than their male counterparts.[36] This gender difference may be driven by unrealistic expectations, family pressure, work-life imbalance, or sleep disorders. Sleep disorders are prevalent among physicians, especially among women, in whom rates are between 35% and 40%.[37,38] The importance of sleep disorders has been emphasized in many studies, which show that changing work schedules, night shifts, and the consecutive fragmented sleep could have a severe cognitive and emotional impact on the performance of physicians on the day after a shift. Independent of gender, the issue of work-life balance has been the subject of great debate and study showing the difficulties of balancing between work and family as important determinants of burnout.[39,40]

The issue of gender would seem to be of particular interest in obstetrics and gynecology, in which now more than 50% of practitioners are women. Despite this obvious need, and the fact that stress reactions and gender have even been studied even among women professional golfers,[41] reports of studies of this aspect of the specialty are conspicuously lacking in the literature.

Workload, a sense of control over one's work environment, and a shared core mission or vision (alignment of core values) were the largest drivers of burnout in a study of practicing primary care physicians.[42] Similarly, a study of transplant surgeons found that unsupportive environments with little decisional control and high work-related demands contribute to the development of burnout.[43]

In general, having some control over schedule and hours worked is associated with reductions in burnout and improved job satisfaction.[44] Professional autonomy, decision-making support and supervision for trainees, and social support have been found to reduce burnout in training programs,[45] but physicians in academic settings tend to have higher rates of burnout.[46] This may not be surprising because the academic environment is more bureaucratic (giving the individual less control), often less efficient, and less able to deal with business matters. Despite this finding, having more control and a reduced workload are not always protective. Well-intentioned efforts to reduce workload, such as the electronic medical records or physician order entry systems, have actually made the problem worse.[47] Even the seeming level of control that comes with being the chairman of a department of obstetrics and gynecology does not reduce burnout rates[48] nor does the resilience of mental health professionals, who one might expect to be able to thwart the threat, who still report burnout rates that approach 25%.[49]

STRESS VERSUS BURNOUT

Stress is often seen as the primary cause of burnout, but there is no single cause of burnout.[8,23] Rather, several factors combine to cause the physical or mental collapse that is burnout. Stress can be a positive or negative factor in our performance. Too little stress leads to feeling underutilized and too much stress leads to collapse from the strain, but there is a middle ground at which stress and expectations maintain focus and peak productivity—deadlines create focus, expectations provide standards to shoot for, and so on. The key is the balance between control and demand: when there is a greater level of control, high demands can be handled. When there is a lack of that control, high demands result in what has been called *toxic stress,* and collapse is likely to occur.

Physically, stress induces the dry mouth, dilated pupils, and the release of adrenalin and noradrenalin associated with the "fight-or-flight" reaction. Psychosocial stress influences cognitive abilities, such as long-term memory retrieval, and has stronger impairing effects on cognitive flexibility in men more than women.[50] In one study, former patients with prolonged work-related stress improved with professional care, but they continued to perform worse than controls after 1 year.[51] In the acute phase, the largest impairments were related to executive function and mental speed, but at follow-up, memory impairments also became apparent.

Burnout, as opposed to stress, is characterized by exhaustion, lack of enthusiasm and motivation, and feelings of ineffectiveness, with the added dimensions of frustration or cynicism, resulting in disengagement, demotivation, and reduced workplace efficacy (**Table 1**). Although chronic stress is identified as one of the key factors, as noted above, no one element is sufficient to exceed the adaptive abilities of the individual. Burnout is generally more gradual, progressive, and insidious than stress, making it more likely to go undetected until further along its continuum.

PERILS OF BURNOUT

Physician burnout is associated with reduced productivity[52] and threatens work-life balance among physicians, especially those in dual career relationships.[1,39] Among emergency physicians, burnout was significantly associated with higher frequencies of self-reported suboptimal care[53] and strongly associated with actual reductions in professional work effort over the following 24 months.[53] Conditions in which there are weak retention rates, high turnover, heavy workloads, low staffing levels, or staffing shortages increase the risk of burnout and, when burnout is present, are associated with a degraded quality of the care provided.[54] Burnout is also associated with an increased risk for physical illness.[55]

Economically, the impact of physician burnout (for physicians practicing in Canada) is estimated to be $213.1 million.[56] This sum includes $185.2 million from early retirement and $27.9 million from reduced clinical hours. In a study of 353 genetic counselors, more than 40% had either considered leaving or left their job role because of burnout.[57] Among residency program directors in radiation oncology surveyed, 11% of respondents met criteria for low burnout, 83% for moderate burnout, and 6% for high burnout. Although 78% of respondents reported feeling "satisfied" or "highly

Table 1
Symptoms of professional burnout

	Early	Midstage	Advanced

Behavioral	Displacement of goals
	Emotional exhaustion:
	  Feeling drained and
	  depleted
	  Starting workdays
	  fatigued
	  No longer look forward
	  to work
	  No longer "bounce
	  back" from time off
	  Working harder
		Depersonalization:
		  Lack of compassion for
		  patients and
		  colleagues
		  More callous toward
		  others
		  Irritable at work
		Denial of emerging
		  problems
		Needless competitive
		  behaviors
		Passive - aggressive
		  behaviors
		  Slow response to pages
		  Skipped meetings
		  Tasks left uncompleted
		  Temper outbursts
			A sense of inner
			  emptiness or
			  exhaustion
			Cynicism
			Depersonalization
			Procrastination

Personal	A compulsion to prove
	  yourself
	Anxiety
	Fatigue not relieved by
	  rest
	Forgetfulness
	Impaired cognitive
	  functions:
	  Short attention span
	  Memory for details is
	  slipping
	  Cognitive rigidity
	Irritability
	Neglecting your own
	  needs
	Poor concentration
		Dread going to work
		Difficulty relaxing or
		  enjoying time off
		Diminished sense of
		  accomplishment:
		  Questioning the value
		  of one's efforts
		  Feeling that nothing
		  has been
		  accomplished
		  Lost the "passion" for
		  work
		Withdrawal
		Worry or anger that
		  contaminates home life
			Apathy
			Depression (including
			  suicidal ideation)
			Withdrawal from
			  friends and family

Physical	Bruxism (Tooth grinding)
	Gastrointestinal problems
	  Headaches
	  Hypertension
	  Insomnia
	  Palpitations
		Chronic sleep
		  disturbances
		Increasing alcohol or
		  other substance use
		More and more intrusive
		  symptoms
			Loss of libido

satisfied" with their current role, 85% planned to remain as program director for less than 5 years.[58]

When advanced, burnout is associated with depression and an increased risk of suicidal ideation. Suicidal ideation has been found to be more prevalent among physicians than in the general population.[59,60] In a meta-analysis, suicide was almost one and a half times more frequent among male physicians compared with the general population and twice as likely for female doctors.[61]

The impact of burnout goes beyond the emotional. Obstetricians must be sensitive to the fact that burnout, whether in patients or female colleagues, is predictor of infertility, miscarriage, and high-risk pregnancy. In a recent study of female Hungarian physicians with burnout, there were more complications of pregnancy, although a clear causal relationship cannot be established[62] despite older studies that found a link between job stress, preterm delivery, and low birth weight for gestational age.[63] Clearly, difficulties achieving, carrying, or delivering a healthy pregnancy themselves are sources of significant stress that could precipitate emotional collapse and burnout for the families involved. There is a great deal of overlap between burnout and other pathologic conditions such as depression,[18] making distinctions between them difficult.

AM I BURNED OUT?

Fatigue and stress are ubiquitous, but that is not the same as burnout. The degree to which the physical, emotional, and professional symptoms are manifest depends on the depth or stage of burnout present (see **Table 1**), making diagnosis problematic. The effective gold standard for diagnosing burnout is the Maslach Burnout Inventory (MBI).[64] The MBI operationalizes burnout as a 3-dimensional syndrome made up of exhaustion, cynicism, and inefficacy. The MBI comprises 3 scales:

1. Emotional exhaustion (9 items), a state of chronic emotional and physical depletion
2. Depersonalization (5 items), a sense of disconnection from coworkers and clients
3. Diminished personal accomplishment (8 items), a negative sense of self-value and ability

Other diagnostic tools have been introduced[65] but have not gained the wide acceptance of the MBI. For example, West and colleagues[66] validated single items from the MBI emotional exhaustion and MBI depersonalization subscales as standalone measures, and this approach has been validated by others.[67] Some investigators have argued that burnout and depression represent different, closely spaced, points along a spectrum and that any effort to separate them may be artificial.[68,69]

Unfortunately, the MBI requires a fee, consists of 22 items, and requires interpretation by a qualified individual. A simpler screening test than the complete MBI consists of 10 screening questions (**Box 1**). If the individual can answer "yes" to 5 or more, they probably have burnout. For most individuals, a simple review of the symptoms and findings found in **Table 1** and **Box 1** will give a reasonable appraisal of the likelihood of burnout. This approach would seem reasonable for simple self-assessment or for broad screening of patients, friends, or family.

Box 1
Burnout screening questions

1. Do you find a lack of pleasure in other activities (anhedonia)?
2. Do you manifest cynicism?
3. Is your work affecting family?
4. Do you dread going to work?
5. Are you easily annoyed?
6. Do you envy those who are happy?
7. Do you no longer care about performance?
8. Do you have fatigue/low energy?
9. Are you bored?
10. Are you depressed before the work week?

Psychologists Herbert Freudenberger and Gail North, studying burnout in women, theorized that the burnout process can be divided into 12 phases.[70] This division has limited utility because the phases are not necessarily followed sequentially, some may be absent, and others may present simultaneously and broadly mimic the symptoms and progression seen in the more general descriptions of characteristics, such as shown in **Table 1**. It is easy to see how a progression of symptoms can represent a potentially spiraling series of behaviors and changes that result in complete dysfunction. It is also easy to understand that the characteristics associated with success in medical school, training, and practice, such as high expectations, placing the needs of others above our own, and a desire to prove oneself, virtually define the first 3 of these stages.

PREVENTION

Because the early symptoms and signs of professional burnout are both common and insidious, prevention and early intervention are always reasonable. Fortunately, there are some simple steps that can be taken to reduce the risk of burnout or to reverse its effects. Because stress and fatigue are 2 of the greatest risk factors for burnout, reducing these is a good place to start. When it comes to fatigue, the solution is easy: sleep. Physicians tend to sleep fewer hours than those in the general population and what is achieved is often not the type that is restful and restorative.[71] Just reducing the number of hours worked is not enough, as several studies have found.[72] The rest must result in relaxation and renewal.

The impact of reduced duty hours might be anticipated to reduce both the fatigue and stress of resident training and, thus, the risk of burnout. In at least 1 study, this has not been the case. In a study of internal medicine residents, year-end burnout prevalence and incidence of burnout did not differ significantly between those before and after the imposition of new work hour restrictions.[73] Interestingly, there was no difference in year-end prevalence of excessive sleepiness (as measured with the Epworth scale) among these same learners. Another study has found that organizations may be able to improve burnout, dissatisfaction, and retention by addressing communication and workflow and initiating quality improvement projects targeting clinician concerns.[74]

Stress reduction may seem more difficult than getting more sleep. Although studies indicate that experience or habituation to stressful situations can blunt the impact of stress,[75] this should not be seen as an adaptive way of dealing with stressful situations. In reality, there are several simple approaches that can be used to reduce stress: alter it (direct communication, problem solving, time management), avoid it (delegate, know limits, walk away), or accept it (build resistance, change perceptions). Even though clinicians all have busy clinical schedules, taking short breaks to rest, sing, laugh, or exercise can go a long way to reducing stress. Shanafelt and colleagues[76] (who have contributed frequently to the burnout literature) found that even breaks as short as 10 minutes can be effective.

Separating work from private life by taking a short break to resolve issues before heading home—avoiding "baggage" or homework—will go a long way to giving perspective from time off. This may also mean that tasks have to be delegated; share chores or get carry out for dinner. Set meaningful, and realistic goals professionally and personally: don't expect or demand more than is possible. This will mean setting priorities—some tasks may have to wait. Finally, don't forget hobbies and activities that are enjoyable.

Physical activity has been shown to reduce feelings of fatigue and provide an improved sense of wellbeing, but this effect appears blunted in the face of chronic

---

Box 2
Burnout prevention and mitigation strategies

Reduce effects
  Health and fitness
  Personal coping strategies
  Rest and relaxation
  Social support

Deal with sources
  Assertiveness
  Be realistic, establish priorities
  Lobby for change
  Time management

Improve attitude
  Highlight the positive
  Let things go
  Look for good
  Reflect and take control

---

stress,[77] limiting its value in reducing the impact of burnout when symptoms are advanced. Paying ourselves with enjoyable activities and hobbies has been shown to promote resiliency.[78]

REVERSING BURNOUT

When symptoms of burnout present, one can reduce the effects, deal with the sources, and improve attitudes (**Box 2**). Rest and relaxation will go a long way to helping, but so will physical wellbeing, a healthy diet, exercise, and health checkups. Dealing with the sources of burnout by identifying the stressors, setting realistic priorities, and time management can also be helpful. Individuals should also lobby for changes that will increase their control and reduce unnecessary obstacles to completing goals. Look for the good and try to identify at least one instance during the day in which your presence or acts made a difference.

Take advantage of mentors, friends, and loved ones to provide perspective, balance, and succor. Because depression and burnout may be virtually indistinguishable,[68,69] seek professional help and counseling early. This help can be in the forms of trained counselors, mentors, clergy, or others. These helpers must be able to respect the individual's privacy and trust but also bring either training or perspective. They can help improve self-awareness and develop coping strategies that are protective. Do not attempt to "go it alone" or self-medicate with antidepressants, alcohol, or other substances—they will only compound the problem.[79]

In the end, obstetricians and gynecologists really do have the tools to reduce, mitigate, or avoid the threat of professional burnout. Just as with the push to include patient satisfaction with any measure of the quality of the medical care we provide, the quality of our own lives must matter. With self-awareness, utilization of coping mechanisms, and reliance on strong social and professional support networks, burnout can be combated.

SUMMARY

The fast pace of life, the impact of multitasking and the unending bombardment of information have made emotional exhaustion almost certain. Studies indicate burnout rates among obstetricians and gynecologists range from 40% to greater than 75%, which places them in the middle to upper third of all specialties. The symptoms of burnout range from feelings of underappreciation and unresolved fatigue to cynicism, depression, and physical symptoms and illness. Burnout is associated with poor job satisfaction, questioning career choices, and dropping out of practice, impacting workforce concerns and patient access.

Awareness of the symptoms and some simple stress and fatigue reduction techniques can reduce the risk of being trapped in the downward spiral of burnout. Awareness of the symptoms of burnout in us, friends, family, and colleagues can allow early diagnosis and intervention. Successful interventions can range from hobbies and vacations to skilled counseling. Whatever the route taken, no physician should feel immune, no physician should feel ashamed or alone, and no physician should feel that reversal is not possible to escape the personal and professional collapse that is burnout.

REFERENCES

1. Shanafelt TD, Boone S, Tan L, et al. Burnout and satisfaction with work-life balance among US physicians relative to the general US population. Arch Intern Med 2012;172(18):1377–85.
2. Martini S, Arfken CL, Churchill A, et al. Burnout comparison among residents in different medical specialties. Acad Psychiatry 2004;28(3):240–2.
3. Medscape Lifestyle Report 2016: Bias and Burnout. Available at: http://www.medscape.com/features/slideshow/lifestyle/2016/public/overview#page=1. Accessed September 16, 2016.
4. Lee YY, Medford AR, Halim AS. Burnout in physicians. J R Coll Physicians Edinb 2015;45(2):104–7.
5. Shanafelt TD, Hasan O, Dyrbye LN, et al. Changes in burnout and satisfaction with work-life balance in physicians and the general US working population between 2011 and 2014. Mayo Clin Proc 2015;90(12):1600–13.
6. Miller N, McGowen R. The painful truth: physicians are not invincible. South Med J 2000;93(10):966–73.
7. Qureshi HA, Rawlani R, Mioton LM, et al. Burnout phenomenon in U.S. plastic surgeons: risk factors and impact on quality of life. Plast Reconstr Surg 2015;135(2):619–26.
8. Streu R, Hansen J, Abrahamse P, et al. Professional burnout among US plastic surgeons: results of a national survey. Ann Plast Surg 2014;72(3):346–50.
9. Evans RW, Ghosh K. A survey of headache medicine specialists on career satisfaction and burnout. Headache 2015;55(10):1448–57.
10. Bragard I, Dupuis G, Fleet R. Quality of work life, burnout, and stress in emergency department physicians: a qualitative review. Eur J Emerg Med 2015;22(4):227–34.
11. Arora M, Asha S, Chinnappa J, et al. Review article: burnout in emergency medicine physicians. Emerg Med Australas 2013;25(6):491–5.
12. Gorelick MH, Schremmer R, Ruch-Ross H, et al. Current workforce characteristics and burnout in pediatric emergency medicine. Acad Emerg Med 2016;23(1):48–54.
13. Garcia TT, Garcia PC, Molon ME, et al. Prevalence of burnout in pediatric intensivists: an observational comparison with general pediatricians. Pediatr Crit Care Med 2014;15(8):e347–53.

14. Shanafelt TD, Balch CM, Bechamps GJ, et al. Burnout and career satisfaction among American surgeons. Ann Surg 2009;250(3):463–71.
15. Rama-Maceiras P, Jokinen J, Kranke P. Stress and burnout in anaesthesia: a real world problem? Curr Opin Anaesthesiol 2015;28(2):151–8.
16. McAbee JH, Ragel BT, McCartney S, et al. Factors associated with career satisfaction and burnout among US neurosurgeons: results of a nationwide survey. J Neurosurg 2015;123(1):161–73.
17. O'Kelly F, Manecksha RP, Quinlan DM, et al. Rates of self-reported 'burnout' and causative factors amongst urologists in Ireland and the UK: a comparative cross-sectional study. BJU Int 2016;117(2):363–72.
18. Wurm W, Vogel K, Holl A, et al. Depression-burnout overlap in physicians. PLoS One 2016;11(3):e0149913.
19. Leung J, Rioseco P, Munro P. Stress, satisfaction and burnout amongst Australian and New Zealand radiation oncologists. J Med Imaging Radiat Oncol 2015;59(1): 115–24.
20. Rath KS, Huffman LB, Phillips GS, et al. Burnout and associated factors among members of the Society of Gynecologic Oncology. Am J Obstet Gynecol 2015; 213(6):824.e1–9.
21. Kawada T. Risk factors of burnout in gynecologic oncologist. Am J Obstet Gynecol 2016;214(4):550–1.
22. Weinstein L. Laborist to obstetrician/gynecologist-hospitalist: an evolution or a revolution? Obstet Gynecol Clin North Am 2015;42(3):415–7.
23. Dyrbye LN, Varkey P, Boone SL, et al. Physician satisfaction and burnout at different career stages. Mayo Clin Proc 2013;88(12):1358–67.
24. IsHak WW, Lederer S, Mandili C, et al. Burnout during residency training: a literature review. J Grad Med Educ 2009;1(2):236–42.
25. Govardhan LM, Pinelli V, Schnatz PF. Burnout, depression and job satisfaction in obstetrics and gynecology residents. Conn Med 2012;76(7):389–95.
26. Becker JL, Milad MP, Klock SC. Burnout, depression, and career satisfaction: cross-sectional study of obstetrics and gynecology residents. Am J Obstet Gynecol 2006;195(5):1444–9.
27. Castelo-Branco C, Figueras F, Eixarch E, et al. Stress symptoms and burnout in obstetric and gynaecology residents. BJOG 2007;114(1):94–8.
28. Parr JM, Pinto N, Hanson M, et al. Medical graduates, tertiary hospitals, and burnout: a longitudinal cohort study. Ochsner J 2016;16(1):22–6.
29. Arora M, Diwan AD, Harris IA. Prevalence and factors of burnout among Australian orthopaedic trainees: a cross-sectional study. J Orthop Surg (Hong Kong) 2014;22(3):374–7.
30. Ogundipe OA, Olagunju AT, Lasebikan VO, et al. Burnout among doctors in residency training in a tertiary hospital. Asian J Psychiatr 2014;10:27–32.
31. Dyrbye LN, West CP, Satele D, et al. Burnout among U.S. medical students, residents, and early career physicians relative to the general U.S. population. Acad Med 2014;89(3):443–51.
32. Thirioux B, Birault F, Jaafari N. Empathy is a protective factor of burnout in physicians: new neuro-phenomenological hypotheses regarding empathy and sympathy in care relationship. Front Psychol 2016;7:763.
33. Lee RT, Seo B, Hladkyj S, et al. Correlates of physician burnout across regions and specialties: a meta-analysis. Hum Resour Health 2013;11:48.
34. Wolf MR, Rosenstock JB. Inadequate sleep and exercise associated with burnout and depression among medical students. Acad Psychiatry 2016. [Epub ahead of print].

35. Kroll HR, Macaulay T, Jesse MA. Preliminary survey examining predictors of burnout in pain medicine physicians in the United States. Pain Physician 2016; 19(5):E689–96.

36. Győrffy Z, Dweik D, Girasek E. Workload, mental health and burnout indicators among female physicians. Hum Resour Health 2016;14:12.

37. Rodrigez-Muñoz A, Moreno-Jimenez B, Fernandez-Mendoza JJ, et al. Insomnia and quality of sleep among primary care physicians: a gender perspective. Rev Neurol 2008;47(3):119–23.

38. Vela-Bueno A, Moreno-Jiménez B, Rodríguez-Muñoz A, et al. Insomnia and sleep quality among primary care physicians with low and high burnout levels. J Psychosom Res 2008;64(4):435–42.

39. Dyrbye LN, Sotile W, Boone S, et al. A survey of U.S. physicians and their partners regarding the impact of work-home conflict. J Gen Intern Med 2014;29(1): 155–61.

40. Roberts DL, Shanafelt TD, Dyrbye LN, et al. National comparison of burnout and work-life balance among internal medicine hospitalists and outpatient general internists. J Hosp Med 2014;9(3):176–81.

41. Kang KD, Hannon JC, Harveson A, et al. Perfectionism and burnout in women professional golfers. J Sports Med Phys Fitness 2016;56(9):1077–85.

42. Gregory ST, Menser T. Burnout among primary care physicians: a test of the areas of worklife model. J Healthc Manag 2015;60(2):133–48.

43. Jesse MT, Abouljoud M, Eshelman A. Determinants of burnout among transplant surgeons: a national survey in the United States. Am J Transplant 2015;15(3): 772–8.

44. Keeton K, Fenner DE, Johnson TR, et al. Predictors of physician career satisfaction, work-life balance, and burnout. Obstet Gynecol 2007;109(4):949–55.

45. Kimo Takayesu J, Ramoska EA, Clark TR, et al. Factors associated with burnout during emergency medicine residency. Acad Emerg Med 2014;21(9):1031–5.

46. Shanafelt TD, Gradishar WJ, Kosty M, et al. Burnout and career satisfaction among US oncologists. J Clin Oncol 2014;32(7):678–86.

47. Shanafelt TD, Dyrbye LN, Sinsky C, et al. Between clerical burden and characteristics of the electronic environment with physician burnout and professional satisfaction. Mayo Clin Proc 2016;91(7):836–48.

48. Gabbe SG, Melville J, Mandel L, et al. Burnout in chairs of obstetrics and gynecology: diagnosis, treatment, and prevention. Am J Obstet Gynecol 2002;186(4): 601–12.

49. Kok BC, Herrell RK, Grossman SH, et al. Prevalence of professional burnout among military mental health service providers. Psychiatr Serv 2016;67(1): 137–40.

50. Shields GS, Trainor BC, Lam JC, et al. Acute stress impairs cognitive flexibility in men, not women. Stress 2016;19(5):542–6.

51. Eskildsen A, Andersen LP, Pedersen AD, et al. Cognitive impairments in former patients with work-related stress complaints - one year later. Stress 2016;19(6): 559–66.

52. Dewa CS, Loong D, Bonato S, et al. How does burnout affect physician productivity? A systematic literature review. BMC Health Serv Res 2014;14:325.

53. Lu DW, Dresden S, McCloskey C, et al. Impact of burnout on self-reported patient care among emergency physicians. West J Emerg Med 2015;16(7):996–1001.

54. Humphries N, Morgan K, Conry MC, et al. Quality of care and health professional burnout: narrative literature review. Int J Health Care Qual Assur 2014;27(4): 293–307.

55. Honkonen T, Ahola K, Pertovaara M, et al. The association between burnout and physical illness in the general population–results from the Finnish Health 2000 Study. J Psychosom Res 2006;61(1):59–66.
56. Dewa CS, Jacobs P, Thanh NX, et al. An estimate of the cost of burnout on early retirement and reduction in clinical hours of practicing physicians in Canada. BMC Health Serv Res 2014;14:254.
57. Johnstone B, Kaiser A, Injeyan MC, et al. The relationship between burnout and occupational stress in genetic counselors. J Genet Couns 2016;25(4):731–41.
58. Aggarwal S, Kusano AS, Carter JN, et al. Stress and burnout among residency program directors in United States radiation oncology programs. Int J Radiat Oncol Biol Phys 2015;93(4):746–53.
59. Tyssen R, Vaglum P, Gronvold NT, et al. Suicidal ideation among medical students and young physicians: a nationwide and prospective study of prevalence and predictors. J Affect Disord 2001;64:69–79.
60. Bernal M, Haro JM, Bernet S, et al. Risk factors for suicidality in Europe: results from the ESEMED study. J Affect Disord 2007;101:27–34.
61. Schernhammer ES, Colditz GA. Suicidal rates among physicians: a quantitative and gender assessment (meta-analysis). Am J Psychiatry 2004;161(12): 2295–302.
62. Győrffy Z, Dweik D, Girasek E. Reproductive health and burn-out among female physicians: nationwide, representative study from Hungary. BMC Womens Health 2014;14:121.
63. Defoe DM, Power ML, Holzman GB, et al. The relation between psychosocial job strain, and preterm delivery and low birthweight for gestational age. Obstet Gynecol 2001;97(6):1015–8.
64. Maslach C, Jackson SE, Leiter MP. MBI: the maslach burnout inventory: manual. Palo Alto (CA): Consulting Psychologists Press; 1996.
65. Kristensen TS, Borritz M, Villadsen E, et al. The Copenhagen Burnout Inventory: a new tool for the assessment of burnout. Work Stress 2005;19:192–207.
66. West C, Dyrbye L, Sloan J, et al. Single item measures of emotional exhaustion and depersonalization are useful for assessing burnout in medical professionals. J Gen Intern Med 2009;24(12):1318–21.
67. Dolan ED, Mohr D, Lempa M, et al. Using a single Item to measure burnout in primary care staff: a psychometric evaluation. J Gen Intern Med 2015;30(5):582–7.
68. Bianchi R, Boffy C, Hingray C, et al. Comparative symptomatology of burnout and depression. J Health Psychol 2013;18(6):782–7.
69. Bianchi R, Schonfeld IS, Laurent E. Is burnout a depressive disorder? A reexamination with special focus on atypical depression. Intl J Stress Mgmt 2014;21(4):307–24.
70. Freudenberger HJ, North G. Women's burnout: how to spot it, how to reverse it, and how to prevent it. Doubleday; 1985.
71. Abrams RM. Sleep deprivation. Obstet Gynecol Clin North Am 2015;42(3): 493–506.
72. Williams D, Tricomi G, Gupta J, et al. Efficacy of burnout interventions in the medical education pipeline. Acad Psychiatry 2015;39(1):47–54.
73. Ripp JA, Bellini L, Fallar R, et al. The impact of duty hours restrictions on job burnout in internal medicine residents: a three-institution comparison study. Acad Med 2015;90(4):494–9.
74. Linzer M, Poplau S, Grossman E, et al. A cluster randomized trial of interventions to improve work conditions and clinician burnout in primary care: results from the Healthy Work Place (HWP) study. J Gen Intern Med 2015;30(8):1105–11.

75. Jezova D, Hlavacova N, Dicko I, et al. Psychosocial stress based on public speech in humans: is there a real life/laboratory setting cross-adaptation? Stress 2016;19(4):429–33.

76. Shanafelt TD, Oreskovich MR, Dyrbye LN, et al. Avoiding burnout: the personal health habits and wellness practices of US surgeons. Ann Surg 2012;255(4): 625–33.

77. Shields GS, Trainor BC, Lam JC, et al. Physical activity buffers fatigue only under low chronic stress. Stress 2016;19(5):535–41.

78. Perez GK, Haime V, Jackson V, et al. Promoting resiliency among palliative care clinicians: stressors, coping strategies, and training needs. J Palliat Med 2015; 18(4):332–7.

79. Cecil J, McHale C, Hart J, et al. Behaviour and burnout in medical students. Med Educ Online 2014;19:25209.

Index

Note: Page numbers of article titles are in **boldface** type.

Obstet Gynecol Clin N Am 44 (2017) 311–320
http://dx.doi.org/10.1016/S0889-8545(17)30061-X
0889-8545/17

obgyn.theclinics.com

Moving?

Make sure your subscription moves with you!

To notify us of your new address, find your **Clinics Account Number** (located on your mailing label above your name), and contact customer service at:

Email: journalscustomerservice-usa@elsevier.com

800-654-2452 (subscribers in the U.S. & Canada)
314-447-8871 (subscribers outside of the U.S. & Canada)

Fax number: 314-447-8029

Elsevier Health Sciences Division
Subscription Customer Service
3251 Riverport Lane
Maryland Heights, MO 63043

*To ensure uninterrupted delivery of your subscription, please notify us at least 4 weeks in advance of move.

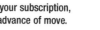

Printed and bound by CPI Group (UK) Ltd, Croydon, CR0 4YY

07/10/2024

01040505-0013